WRITING AND READING
MENTAL HEALTH RECORDS

Issues and Analysis in
Professional Writing and
Scientific Rhetoric
Second Edition

WRITING AND READING MENTAL HEALTH RECORDS
Issues and Analysis in
Professional Writing and
Scientific Rhetoric
Second Edition

John Frederick Reynolds
City College of CUNY

David C. Mair
University of Oklahoma, Norman

Pamela C. Fischer
Private Practice, Oklahoma City

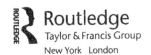
Routledge
Taylor & Francis Group
New York   London

First published by Lawrence Erlbaum Associates, Inc., Publishers
10 Industrial Avenue
Mahwah, New Jersey 07430

Transferred to digital printing 2010 by Routledge

Routledge

270 Madison Avenue
New York, NY 10016

2 Park Square, Milton Park
Abingdon, Oxon OX14 4RN, UK

Library of Congress Cataloging-in-Publication Data

Reynolds, John Frederick, 1952-
   Writing and reading mental health records: issues and analysis in
   professional writing and scientific rhetoric, second edition /   John
Frederick Reynolds, David C. Mair, Pamela C. Fischer.
         p.   cm.
      Includes bibliographical references and index.
      ISBN 0-8058-2001–9(c : alk paper). -- ISBN 0-8058-2002-7
   (alk. paper)
      1. Psychiatric records.   2. Psychiatric hospitals--Re-
   cords.
      I. Mair, David Clare, 1949-   .   II.   Fischer, Pamela C.
   (Pamela Correia) III. Title.
      RC455.2.M38R49 1995
      616.89′0751--dc20   95-19440
                                                  CIP

10 9 8 7 6 5 4 3 2 1

Contents

A Rhetorician's Foreword

Lee Odell
Rensselaer Polytechnic Institute

Mental health reports? What a strange thing for composition specialists to be concerned with. These reports are filled with a jargon that is inaccessible to composition teachers and that is even misinterpreted by mental health professionals. These reports don't really constitute a definable genre (the authors of this text caution that their own efforts to define the genre, as reflected in their Taxonomy in chapter 2, probably cannot be generalized beyond the settings where they did their research). And it is hard to see how understanding these reports would contribute to the teaching of composition—at least to anyone other than mental health professionals. So why mental health reports?

As it happens, *Writing and Reading Mental Health Records* presents a series of rather compelling answers to this question. The first is that these reports are important because, directly or indirectly, they will touch virtually everyone's life. The authors note that at least one in five Americans will probably, at some point in their lives, seek treatment for a mental disorder. And those who do not seek treatment for themselves will be affected by those who do—friends, family, and significant others, not to mention all sorts of adult and juvenile criminal offenders. For all these persons, the mental health report will be the basis for answering such questions as these: Is this person in fact suffering from a treatable mental disorder? If so, what sort of treatment should the person receive? Will an insurance company have to reimburse him or her for that treatment? Is the treatment succeeding? Should this person be held legally responsible for his or her actions? As a society and as individuals, we have reason to care about answers to these questions.

Second, these reports may present an opportunity for us to do something useful in the world outside our classrooms. This is not to suggest we should go barging in to mental health organizations advocating features of diction, syntax, or organization that have always served us well in our teaching and in our own writing. Quite the contrary. As this book makes clear, when we enter a particular mental health setting, we are strangers in a land that may be quite different from what we are accustomed to, maybe even different from other mental health settings. As the authors point out, perhaps the most consistent feature of mental health reports is their extreme variability.

But our status as outsiders may stand us in good stead. If we can rein in our teacherly impulse to jump in and propose solutions before we know exactly what the problems are, our lack of understanding can enable mental health professionals to surface their assumptions and tacit knowledge, and then subject both knowledge and assumptions to scrutiny or revision. Our lack of knowledge can be an occasion for them to teach us and themselves as well. And it can let us find points at which the things we do know—as writers, as teachers of writing—can be useful. Once we understand the values and goals of a given setting, we can use what we know about diction, syntax, organization, or the composing process to help people achieve these goals.

And finally, mental health reports are important to teachers of writing because they constitute, in the authors' words, "practitioner rhetorics," and, as such, occasions to test and refine our assumptions about the ways meaning gets constructed and conveyed through language. Consider, for example, just one of the several types of writing done in medical mental health settings—the nursing assessment. This assessment, written within 24 hours after a patient has been admitted to a mental health hospital, obliges a nurse to develop a comprehensive understanding of "the patient's physical, mental, and spiritual condition." The nurse has to use that understanding to determine what the patient's problems are, set up goals, and propose "immediate interventions" that will help achieve these goals. This assessment may be read by any number of people—physician, pastoral counselor, social worker, occupational/recreational therapist—and it becomes part of the basis for setting up the patient's "master treatment plan."

By any standard, this is a formidable rhetorical task. It also is an opportunity for us to think through such questions as these: What "ideological biases" (see chapter 3) are reflected in the language the nurse/rhetorician uses to talk to and talk about the patient? What details do those biases predispose him or her to see? To ignore? In other words, how does language figure into the process of constructing meaning in this context? What social interactions—with the patient, with other nurses, with physicians—influence the nurse's attempt to construct meaning in this context? And how do readers of the assessment construct their own meanings of the assessment?

These are the kinds of questions this book will help us answer, not by addressing them directly but by providing a map of an extraordinarily complex territory. Particularly valuable in this respect are the authors' discussions of the language of mental health reports and the "ideological biases" that govern the work of mental health professionals. These discussions help us see what kinds of questions can and should be asked. By enabling us to investigate the language and thought of one type of nonacademic setting, this book enables us to consider issues that are fundamental to our field.

Why think about mental health reports? *That's* why.

A Clinician's Foreword

James L. Levenson
Medical College of Virginia

When I was a third-year medical student, during my first experiences in patient care, a wise old medical resident told me that, contrary to what I had been taught, the patient interview and physical examination were not the most important parts of patient assessment. He proclaimed that 90% of what we needed to know about a new patient could be found in the old chart. He was often proved right. Despite its critical importance, the role of the patient record in clinical management has remained largely unexamined. This is especially ironic in mental health care, because psychiatrists and other mental health professionals have traditionally placed great emphasis on the value of constructing a narrative account of the patient's history, tracing a life from its prenatal start through key phases of development, major traumas, significant relationships, past and present symptoms, and up to the present illness or problem.

Although we mental health professionals read, photocopy, fax, and often obsess over the content of our clinical records, we seldom consider their structure, format, language, or process of construction. Why should that be? *Writing and Reading Mental Health Records* provides us insight because its first two authors are teachers of composition, specialists in technical and professional writing, working in collaboration with a psychologist. For all our uses of language and persuasion, we in the mental health professions are not expert in linguistics or rhetoric. As the authors of this book diplomatically note, we are unaware of many issues regarding our records because we have never been trained to be aware of them.

But there are other explanations, as well, that can account not only for our inattention to the form and process of our records, but also for a deterioration in their focus and quality of content. The authors of *Writing and Reading Mental Health Records* remind us of the increasingly powerful influences of various institutions and social forces on how mental health records are written. Rapidly changing health care-delivery systems, third-party payors, the Joint Commission on Accreditation of Hospitals (JCAH), malpractice suits, federal and state regulations—all have had a tremendous impact on mental health care and how it is recorded. Each has had obvious as well as subtle and occult effects on how the encounter between the mental health professional and the patient is recorded. Unfortunately, the influences do not easily integrate with each other or with our primary purpose, treating the patient. No wonder, then, that the mental health record has become a bewildering quilt of different professional jargons and bureaucratic imperatives. No wonder we may even lose sight of the readers for whom our records are written. No wonder that a composition specialist might look on the mental health delivery system as a Tower of Babel.

This book and its authors have raised many questions for me. To what extent do initial impressions recorded on intake records distort subsequent diagnostic assessment and treatment planning? That is, if the initial impressions are erroneous in some major way, how often are the errors perpetuated by uncritical acceptance? To what extent does record-keeping differ between settings (state hospital vs. private hospital, outpatient fee-for-service vs. outpatient HMO, etc.)? What is the relationship between the characteristics of records and reimbursement? Are there differences between the records of Medicare, Medicaid, Blue Cross/Blue Shield, private insurance, and indigent patients? How is reimbursement affected by the structure, content, and process of records? Can we develop meaningful quality standards for records beyond externally mandated standards (e.g., JCAH)? How far have our conscious and unconscious responses to the fear of malpractice suits distorted our record-keeping?

Reynolds, Mair, and Fischer have brought new light to where we stand in our clinical work. I hope this book stimulates your thinking as much as it has mine.

Preface to the Second Edition

Words were originally magic and to this day have retained much of their ancient magical power. By words one person can make another blissfully happy or drive him to despair ... convey his knowledge ... carry his audience with him and determine their judgments and decisions.

—Sigmund Freud
The Introductory Lectures

Writing and Reading Mental Health Records, Second Edition, is a rhetorical analysis of written communication in the mental health community. As such, it contributes to the growing body of research being done these days in rhetoric and composition studies on the nature of writing and reading in highly specialized professional discourse communities.

At least since the landmark work of scholars Odell and Goswami (1982, 1985), professional writing in nonacademic settings has been a subject of interest to postsecondary rhetoric and composition studies specialists. As Matalene (1989) observed in her important book, *Worlds of Writing: Teaching and Learning in Discourse Communities of Work*, rhetoric and composition specialists in university English departments have increasingly recognized the importance of studying all uses of language, not just literary uses; of offering direction and insight to all users of English, not just to freshmen and poets and literary critics; of building better bridges between the academy and the public; of learning and teaching in the many worlds of writing other than their own. Similarly, professionals from various worlds of work have increasingly begun to realize that to be a white-collar worker today very much means to be a writer; that whether one's actual profession be law, accounting, medicine, engineering, management, or whatever, it is to some extent the profession of writing.

As a result, writing specialists in university English departments are now often entering into research partnerships with colleagues from other academic disciplines so that various worlds of technical, professional, and scientific writing can be examined from an interdisciplinary perspective. Both editions of *Writing and Reading Mental Health Records* resulted from one such interdisciplinary research partnership, in this particular case an ongoing collaboration between composition studies specialists and mental health practitioners. This book has always been imagined as being a book by and for both groups, a book that might present research of value not only to writing scholars and teachers, but also to professional clinicians, their teachers, and those who read mental health records in order to make critically important decisions. As Scholes (1991) noted, "Because of the importance and power of [scientific] discourses it is essential for students to learn how they work and what their strengths, costs, and limitations may be" (p. 11).

One of the most complex worlds of writing in our society (we continue to believe that it is, in fact, the most complex world) is the mental health community, a community of professional writers and readers who depend on a plethora of documents full of careful description, interpretation, and analysis for informed and intelligent decision making. Like those writers and readers, we intend to be both descriptive and interpretive in the rhetorical analysis that follows. Our purposes are to describe, interpret, and analyze the nature of written communication in the mental health community; to bring to life many of the major terms, concepts, and theories currently at the center of postsecondary rhetoric and composition studies; to suggest, at least implicitly, one model for further book-length studies of professional writing communities; and to offer insights that might be used to improve writing and its instruction in the world of mental health. In the case of the latter, we believe our research indicates that much is at stake.

Psychiatrists, psychologists, social workers, nurses, therapists, counselors; lawyers, judges, caseworkers, parole boards, probation officers; classroom teachers, school psychologists, guidance counselors—all of those professionals who for one reason or another currently do or someday will write and/or read mental health records need to do so with the greatest possible caution and care. All need the fullest possible awareness of the complexities and political realities of rhetorical situation(s). The writers need the greatest possible understanding of the tensions and complications that result when almost everything they write will have multiple audiences, purposes, and uses. The readers need the greatest possible consciousness of the fact that almost everything they read probably resulted from complex acts of "discovery, negotiation, compromise, commitment, creation, persuasion, and control" (Matalene, 1989, p. xi). We have always hoped that *Writing and Reading Mental Health Records*, in its various editions, would help to start dialogues that over time might meet some of these needs.

Our work on mental health records had its beginnings in a 1987–1988 research study that we conducted in Oklahoma with the ongoing assistance of Robert Edwards, Mark Hayes, Terri Goodman, Daina Baker, John Holter, Judy Norlin, Donna Johnson, Thomas Miller, the staffs of North Care Center and Bethany Pavilion, and Oklahoma Mental Health Commissioner L. Frank James. Preliminary results from that study were published in 1989 in the *Journal of Technical Writing and Communication*, and we appreciate Baywood Publishing Company's permission to reprint much of that material here in chapter 2.

We gratefully acknowledge the hundreds of professional writer-clinicians whose names we can never know but whose work has made both book-length expansions of that original study possible. We are enormously indebted to the dozens of colleagues who have granted us lengthy interviews, answered our follow-up questions, made important suggestions, and/or offered comments, sometimes anonymously, for inclusion in both editions of our book. We appreciate the invaluable help we have received from Dale R. Fuqua, Lodema Correia, and Cindy Gregory, as well as the many hours Warden Jack Cowley has allowed us to spend interviewing staff and observing activities at the Joseph Harp Correctional Center.

I personally want to thank Ann A. Hohmann of the National Institute of Mental Health (NIMH) for her many useful insights, and for putting me in touch with James L. Levenson, who has been enormously helpful to us on more than one occasion over the years. Karen Bourdon, also of NIMH, needs to be acknowledged for her patience in responding to my dumb, no doubt, but critically important questions about the Epidemiologic Catchment Area study. I want to publicly express my appreciation to Marquita Flemming of Sage Publications, and to the many kind reviewers of our first edition—Nancy Comley, Robert McDonald, Carolyn Matalene, and Carol Reeves, in particular—for their support. Also those colleagues who wrote letters nominating our first edition for the NCTE award for Best Book on Technical or Scientific Writing for 1992.

I must once again acknowledge my former department chair, linguist Charles E. Ruhl, a remarkable human being who always understood, as Freud understood, the magical power of words, and who unfailingly used his most magical words to support the early stages of this, and other, work during my years on the faculty of Old Dominion University, where support was often long on talk and short on do. But most of all I want to thank three people: my wacky psychologist father-in-law, Robert Edwards, for introducing me to his fascinating world of work and to my friend and colleague Pamela Fischer; my long-time cohort and collaborator, David Mair, whose words, phrases, clauses, ideas, suggestions, questions, objections, and reactions are, for me, always so incredibly useful and perfectly on-target that I find myself reaching for the phone even when I have no real reason for calling; and my editor at Lawrence Erlbaum Associates, Hollis Heimbouch, who has faithfully and enthusiastically supported not only my work, but the work of many people in rhetoric and composition studies, and with whom I would be proud to work together on anything, anytime, anywhere.

—*Fred Reynolds*

The truth of everything and all people after Plato is writing: you are, one might say, either what you write down, or what somebody else writes down about you.

—Jasper Neel
Plato, Derrida, and Writing
1988

Introduction

THE GROWING IMPORTANCE OF MENTAL HEALTH RECORDS

We should never forget that John Tower was denied the chance to be George Bush's Secretary of State [sic] because there were records of his alcoholism, or that Thomas Eagleton was denied the chance to be George McGovern's running mate because there were records of his shock therapy, or that Richard Nixon was denied the chance to be President because there were some psychiatric records he wanted from some safe in an office at the Watergate Hotel.

—Anonymous Psychiatrist in Private Practice

Problems associated with writing and reading mental health records are well worth our attention. Large and ever-increasing numbers of people are going to be affected by the writing and reading of these records sometime during their lifetimes. As we approach the 21st century, more and more people are entering into an increasing number of mental health care-delivery systems. At the same time, growing numbers of problems are coming to be defined as mental disorders. Consequently, increasing numbers of people are writing and reading increasing numbers of mental health records for increasing numbers of purposes, and that trend is likely to continue.

Lewis L. Judd (1990), former director of the National Institute of Mental Health (NIMH), pointed out that mental disorders are much more common than most people realize. They are hardly rare, he explained, and they do not happen only to others. Schizophrenia, for example, one of the less common mental disorders, is 5 times more common than multiple sclerosis, 6 times more common than insulin-dependent diabetes, and 60 times more common than muscular dystrophy.

Overall, NIMH epidemiologic research has suggested that mental health disorders have a prevalence in the general population about that of hypertension, and thus significant numbers of people are at risk for mild to severe impairments

1

(Freedman, 1984). In fact, one in every five Americans will have a mental disorder at some time in life (according to one study, the number may be as high as one in three), and one in five will seek treatment (Judd, 1990; Regier, Boyd, Burke, Rae, & Myers, 1988).

Society's thinking, as well as the mental health community's thinking, about what constitutes *mental illness* and *treatment* has changed dramatically during the past two decades. Definitions of both terms have expanded significantly. This has been especially true for alcohol and other drug abuse and dependency, now readily defined as mental disorders and treated as such. A variety of other codependent, addictive, or otherwise dysfunctional human behaviors are now seen as mental disorders as well. To the extent that such things as chemical dependency, eating disorders, domestic violence, and post-traumatic stress disorders (PTSDs), for example, have only relatively recently come to be thought of by large segments of the public and the clinical community as mental disorders rather than weaknesses of will, the already dramatic mental illness statistics and trends may reveal only the tip of an iceberg of mental illness in our society at the turn of the century.

Before we look at some of those statistics and trends, we think it is important to note just how fluid and interactive the mental health care "system" is. For example, we believe that the stigma-reducing "treatable disorder" movement during the last two decades has enormous implications which the overall system has only barely begun to realize, especially when that particular movement interacts with insurance carriers' responses to it. Consider the following chain reaction: Once a given problem comes to be seen as a treatable disorder, more people begin to seek treatment for that disorder, causing more documents to be generated. More people begin to be documented, in writing, as having had that disorder, as having been treated for it, successfully or unsuccessfully. But as the demand for treatment of that disorder under health insurance coverage begins to increase, insurance companies begin to impose limits on coverage. (We should note here that mental health care is perhaps the easiest health insurance coverage category, politically, in which to cut benefits. As a recent article on psychiatric hospital insurance problems noted, "Because of the relative imprecision of mental illness diagnosis, it is easier for insurers to challenge psychiatric admissions than admissions for other ailments. In many cases, insurers are simply decreasing the limits on psychiatric inpatient stays, no matter what a doctor prescribes," "Psychiatric Hospitals," 1991.) In reponding to these constantly changing coverage limits, then, the clinical community feels it has no real choice but to constantly change, as well; that is, to keep developing alternative definitions of illness and approaches to treatment so that clinicians can receive payment for services. Our point here is that the entire situation is remarkably fluid, and likely to become increasingly so. Written documentation plays a key role, of course, in that fluidity. Under current definitions of illness and treatment, mental health records already affect many, many people; and as definitions expand, written records will begin to affect even more.

THE MENTAL HEALTH PICTURE TODAY:
A THUMBNAIL SKETCH

The following is a thumbnail sketch of the national mental health picture as of the mid-1990s—current definitions of *disorder, treatment,* and selected current trends and statistics. Although the latter are not complete in their coverage, not a mental health status report per se, they do suggest the growing importance of mental health records in our society.

Current Definitions of Disorder

Current editions of the American Psychiatric Association's *Diagnostic and Statistical Manual of Mental Disorders* (the *DSM*) officially recognize, name, define, and describe more than 40 mental illnesses, 15 of them major, according to the following general categories:

- infant, childhood, or adolescent disorders
- organic mental disorders
- substance abuse disorders
    alcohol
    drugs
- schizophrenic disorders
- paranoid disorders
- psychotic disorders
- affective disorders
    mania
    depression
    dysthymia
- anxiety disorders
    phobias
    panic
    obsessive-compulsive disorders
- somatoform disorders
- dissociative disorders
- psychosexual disorders
- factitious disorders
- impulse control disorders
- adjustment disorders
- other and additional

Current Definitions of Treatment

The following are currently considered to be among the major mental health care treatment settings, at least for purposes of NIMH utilization studies (Shapiro, Skinner, Kessler, Von Korff, & German, 1984):

Specialty Mental Health Resources

- Psychiatrists, psychologists, social workers, other counselors working in private practice or family clinics
- Mental health centers
- Psychiatric hospitals, and psychiatric units of general medical hospitals
- Outpatient clinics at psychiatric hospitals
- Drug treatment clinics
- Alcohol treatment clinics

General Medical Resources

- Medical care practitioners to whom visits are made for emotional or mental problems

Other Resources

- School counseling services
- Prison counseling services
- Church and other pastoral counseling services
- Family service agencies
- Crisis centers, women's centers, etc.

Current Trends and Statistics

At present, the most common mental illnesses are the anxiety disorders (phobias, panic, and obsessive-compulsive disorder) and the affective disorders (depression, manic-depression, and dysthymia; Regier et al., 1988). Men currently have higher rates of diagnosis for the substance abuse and antisocial personality disorders, whereas women currently have higher rates of diagnosis for the affective, anxiety, and somatization disorders (Regier et al., 1988). Higher prevalence rates for most of the disorders are currently found among people below age 45 (Regier et al., 1988). But those rates may change as the population ages: Psychiatric conditions tend to be exacerbated by the stress of chronic and multiple physical illness that accompany aging; and for at least 5% of those over age 65, cognitive deficits or dementia occurs, with associated changes in behavior and affect (Bender, 1990).

Medication decisions are often based upon a written history of the patient's prior responses. Without this history, the selection of one agent over another in its pharmacologic class is more often guided by adverse reaction rates than by a knowledge of which agent will be the most effective for the patient.

—Kenneth J. Bender, PharmD
Psychiatric Pharmacologist

Mental disorders appear to be interrelated. Currently, there is a "general tendency toward co-occurrence, so that the presence of any disorder increase[s] the odds of having another disorder" (Boyd, Burke, Gruenberg, Holzer, & Rae, 1984, p. 983). In certain cases, the tendency toward co-occurrence is dramatic. NIMH research has shown, for example, "that a pre-existing anxiety disorder or major depressive episode among people 18 to 30 years of age *doubles the risk for future substance abuse and dependence*" (Judd, 1990; italics added). Alcohol and drug abuse/dependency and mental illness appear to be especially interdependent. Up to 53% of drug abusers and 37% of alcoholics have at least one serious mental illness. Similarly, 29% of all mentally ill people have a problem with either alcohol or drug abuse (Bass, 1990). Given the tendency toward interrelationship and co-occurrence of mental illnesses, then, we should consider, at the very least, the current and future systemic significance of the following.

Alcoholism.   At present, the magnitude and consequences of alcoholism are enormous. An estimated 10 to 20 million people in the United States are alcoholics (Bender, 1990; McGrath, Kelta, Strickland, & Russo, 1990; Steele & Josephs, 1990). Alcohol consumption contributes to 1 out of every 10 deaths in the United States, approximately 200,000 each year (Bender, 1990). Alcohol abuse is implicated in 70% of fatal automobile accidents, 65% of murders, 88% of knifings, 65% of spouse batterings, 55% of child abuse, 60% of burglaries (Steele & Josephs, 1990), and somewhere between 20% and 37% of suicides (McGrath et al., 1990). No other psychoactive substance is associated with violent crimes, suicide, and automobile accidents more than alcohol (Steele & Josephs, 1990). Alcohol abuse is currently the nation's most costly health problem: "When the costs of lost production, crime, and accidents due to alcohol are totaled and added to the cost of treating alcohol addiction, the bill comes to over $117 billion a year" (Steele & Josephs, 1990, p. 921).

The devastation of alcoholism, as with other drug abuse, can also be measured in terms of the destruction of the individual's self-worth, relationships, and the emotional health of associated family, friends, and coworkers (Bender, 1990). Thirty to 50% of the alcoholics in the country today are women, for whom alcoholism leads to increased rates of pancreatitis, cirrhosis, ulcers, and cardiovascular problems. Many women use alcohol to repress traumatic childhood experiences including sexual and physical abuse and incest (McGrath et al., 1990). Although the evidence suggests that some forms of alcoholism have a significant genetic basis, environmentally induced processes have the most powerful influence on the development of alcoholism, and "thus behavioral psychology enters the picture" (Steele & Josephs, 1990, pp. 928–929).

Abuse of Other Drugs.   Illicit drug abuse is pervasive in U.S. society. It is widely believed by many experts in the field that the level of drug abuse in the United States is higher than that in any other industrialized nation (National Institute on Drug Abuse [NIDA], 1989). More than one half of U.S. youth try an illicit drug before they finish high school. An estimated 14.5 million Americans used a drug illicitly in the month prior to being surveyed in the 1988 National

Household Survey on Drug Abuse (NIDA, 1989). The number of people admitted to emergency rooms following cocaine use increased more than fivefold since 1990. The number of people who died following cocaine use more than doubled during the same time period (NIDA, 1989).

Drug abuse in the United States is clearly a major public health problem. In addition to medical emergencies and deaths related to drug abuse, other short- and long-term effects have been identified: automobile accidents, workplace accidents, learning disabilities, interference with reproduction, fetal injury, and long-term damage to heart, lungs, and other organs (NIDA, 1989). The U.S. Department of Health and Human Services' (U.S. DHHS) 1990 National Household Survey on Drug Abuse showed declining use of most illicit drugs by Americans. Despite the apparent good news, however, drug abuse remained high among members of key demographic subgroups: young adults ages 18–25, African Americans, individuals in large cities, and the unemployed. According to former Health and Human Services Secretary Louis Sullivan, drug abuse continues to account for a significant portion of the violence, crime, child abuse, and other destructive behaviors in our society (U.S. DHHS, 1990).

Teenage Depression and Suicide.   Suicide is correlated with depression in adolescents. Approximately 5,000 young people commit suicide each year, with as many as 300,000 to 400,000 attempts every year in the general population (McGrath et al., 1990). Since the 1960s, the suicide rates for young people have almost tripled. In addition, adolescent suicides are often followed by a "cluster" effect in which one suicide is followed by other attempts (and some completions) from young people in the same community (McGrath et al., 1990).

According to a recent Gallup poll, 6% of U.S. teenagers say that they have tried to commit suicide, and 15% say that they have come close to trying. Three out of five surveyed said that they knew a teenager who had attempted suicide; 15% said that they knew a teenager who had succeeded. Almost 33% of those surveyed said that the suicidal teenager had exhibited warning signs, such as depression or withdrawal, or had talked or written about wanting to die. Of those teens who reported having considered or attempted suicide, 47% blamed family problems, 23% cited depression, 22% cited problems with friends, 18% cited feeling worthless, and 16% cited boy–girl relationships. Some gave more than one reason. The senior analyst for the survey, a former school psychologist, commented that the poll proved that society had not addressed one of its major problems: "The third largest cause of death among adolescents is suicide," he reported, "and yet you don't really see anybody systematically addressing this yet" ("6% of Teens Say, 1991).

According to a study published in the June 1991 issue of *Pediatrics*, a major portion of teen suicides and suicide attempts can be attributed to homosexual and bisexual males. The study reported that nearly one third of all gay male teenagers attempt suicide at least once, suggesting "an urgent public health problem warranting further study" (Majeski, 1991).

Homelessness. Homelessness in the United States continues to increase, and interrelationships between alcoholism, drug abuse, mental illness, and homelessness seem clear (Rossi, 1990). In the mid-1950s, there were more than 550,000 patients in U.S. public mental health hospitals. Now there are about 100,000. Almost one third of the homeless in New York City alone—about 15,000—are mentally ill persons who would have been in hospital-based treatment in the 1960s (Rosenthal, 1990). Estimates of the rates of mental illness among the homeless vary widely, from about 10% to more than 85%, but most studies report rates on the order of 33%, an increase from estimated rates appearing in the literature of the 1950s and 1960s (Rossi, 1990).

Post-Traumatic Stress Disorders. Post-traumatic stress disorder (PTSD), what Menninger once described as a "whiplash of the soul," was originally associated primarily with military combat and was not officially recognized as a bonafide mental disorder until 1980, long enough after the Vietnam War had ended that most Vietnam-related cases of PTSD likely saw delayed treatment or no treatment at all. Today, however, combat-related PTSD may loom large on the mental health horizon. It is feared by some, for example, that an especially large number of the more than 500,000 troops sent to the Persian Gulf in 1990–1991 (as well as many of their parents, spouses, and children) will enter into mental health care-delivery systems over the next few years for treatment of nightmares, depression, substance abuse, and relationship troubles that may have resulted from stresses associated with their military service (Pate, 1991).

Furthermore, PTSD diagnoses are no longer being linked solely to military or combat-related experiences. The physical, cognitive, and behavioral responses of female sexual abuse and assault victims, for example, are now seen as as being consistent with *DSM* criteria for PTSD (Koss, 1990). In fact, some experts consider female sexual abuse and assault victims to be the largest single group of PTSD sufferers, and believe the size of that group is huge and likely to increase. When epidemiologic methods have been applied to the study of violence against women, the results suggest that sexual abuse and assault have been experienced by 38% to 67% of adult women recalling the period before age 18, 12% of adolescent girls, 15% of college women, and approximately 20% of adult women. In addition, violence in the recent relationships is reported by 31% of married women. Alarmingly, "all of the studies document levels of violence that far outdistance office estimates. They suggest a scourge of violence against women in the United States" (Koss, 1990, p. 375).

Clinical recognition of PTSD and other mental disorders in adult female victims of violence is thus on the rise. Even when evaluated many years after an assault, victims are significantly more likely than nonvictims to qualify for psychiatric diagnoses of major depression, alcohol and/or drug abuse or dependence, generalized anxiety, obsessive-compulsive disorder, and PTSD (Koss, 1990). Increasingly, victimization in general is being recognized as a significant etiology in eating disorders, multiple personality, and borderline syndrome. It is now "abundantly clear that a history of victimization is a strong risk factor for development of lifetime mental health problems" (Koss, 1990, p. 376).

Other "New Mental Health Disorders." Just as chemical dependency and PTSD only recently received widespread acknowledgment as mental disorders, as bonafide mental illnesses, other "new mental health disorders" are constantly in the process of being identified, recognized, and accepted by both the public and mental health community. Some are quite technical (e.g., Late Luteal Phase Dyspheric Disorder), whereas others are simply faddish. One regional magazine, for example, recently published a special issue exploring

> some mental health disorders [*sic*] just now coming out of the closet and being recognized as warranting specialized treatment: difficult children, problems with intimacy, co-addictive behavior, adults molested as children, looking for father, toilet training, facing infertility, talking man to man, family trauma, addictive relapse. (*Fourth Annual Guide*, 1990, p. 1)

These, and others, may soon come to be seen as mental health disorders, prompting large numbers of people to seek treatment.

CONCLUSION

The long-term U.S. mental health picture, then, is likely to be one of rising incidence and prevalence of a growing number of disorders and associated disorders, leading to an increasing number of patients entering into an increasing number of care-delivery systems, where more mental health records will be written, read, kept, and utilized. From a records point of view, the mental health picture resonates with paradox. Given the enormously destructive social and economic effects of mental illness, it is critical that more of the mentally ill seek treatment, that more be diagnosed and treated effectively in as many settings as necessary, and that (if necessary) more be covered by insurance and other third-party payment sources so that care can be made available to them. However, as more people are treated for mental health problems, more become dependent on and vulnerable to mental health records. Records play a critical systemic role, and the larger the system, the larger the role of the records.

Compared to other mental health issues, however, the records are a largely unexplored aspect of the mental health care picture in the United States, despite their obvious importance both now and in the future to the increasing numbers of patients, practioners, and third parties who collectively comprise the mental health care system.

For patients, written records facilitate the delivery and, perhaps, determine the quality of mental health care services. They certainly facilitate and determine levels of reimbursement when insurance coverage is involved. And because they become part of patients' life histories, mental health records can come back to save and, as well, to haunt.

For practitioners, written records play an important role in a wide variety of care-delivery contexts. They facilitate and determine levels of payment for services when insurance coverage is involved. Because they become part of practitioners' decision-making histories, mental health records can come back to protect and, as well, to expose.

For third parties, written records are equally important. Employers, educators, insurance companies, government agencies, professional organizations, and others regularly rely on mental health documentation when making decisions, gathering data, assessing needs, allocating resources, and formulating policies.

As one final indicator of the importance of mental health records in our society, we could consider for a moment their use by the courts, one especially powerful third party in the U.S. mental health picture. There can be no doubt that courts use mental health evaluations for important decision-making purposes. For all who seek treatment, either now or in the future, either voluntarily or involuntarily, by today's definitions of illness or tomorrow's, diagnoses will be made and documents will be written and read. Were those records used for no other purposes, in no other contexts, they would be well worth studying for their legal implications alone.

Early in my career I was not lawsuit-conscious. But after a few experiences with hungry attorneys, I soon became very lawsuit-conscious whenever I made a written entry in any record.

—Marcia Haynes, RNC, CHSA
Correctional Health Services Administrator

Every single day, in such judicial and quasi-judicial contexts as sentencing, parole, child custody, disability, and inheritance proceedings, mental health records are used by real people making real decisions affecting real people's lives. As American Psychological Association (APA) past-president Joseph D. Matarazzo (1990) noted:

Society has accorded professional psychologists the privileged status of expert witness. As such we are involved in human dramas and in decisions that are extremely costly not only to the humans involved but also to insurance companies and other segments of society, which pay the millions of dollars juries award, often because of the expert testimony psychologists have contributed. (p. 1003)

In today's personal-injury-initiated psychological-assessment consultations, large sums of money are involved. It is not unusual for a clinical psychologist or clinical neuropsychologist to examine, at the request of an attorney, insurance company, or other payer, a person who alleges brain injury or a stress disorder and whose request for redress involves millions of dollars. Psychologists are no longer examining only the school child who appears to be a slow learner; the healthy child in a custody battle, as well as each parent, have also become the focus of examination. (p. 1002)

These records, in other words, matter.

Chapter 1

A Review of the Literature on Mental Health Records

We spend countless hours teaching graduate psychology students and psychiatric residents how to interview, how to administer and interpret tests, and how to do therapy. All of these enterprises end up on paper. ... And yet there is little or no training given on how to write.

—Jack T. Huber
Report Writing in Psychology and Psychiatry
1961

INTRODUCTION AND OVERVIEW: FROM THE 1940s TO THE 1990s

Problems associated with writing and reading mental health records have been a subject of concern among both scholars and clinicians since the 1940s. In this chapter, we review in detail what we believe to be the key contributions to the professional literature on mental health records to date. We think it might be useful to preface our review by calling special attention to several themes that consistently recur throughout this body of literature:

Theme 1: There has been relatively little systematic study of mental health records, despite the critical role they play in patient care and management.

Theme 2: Mental health practitioners receive surprisingly little training in how to write and read a record, given the amount of time they tend to spend doing both.

Theme 3: Communication between professionals in the mental health community is especially complicated as a result of its unusually wide variety of writer/reader backgrounds, care-delivery settings, and documentation standards.

The following two studies, for example, were published more than four decades apart, and yet they focus on the same basic findings:

In 1946, **Taylor and Teicher**[1] reported in the *Journal of Clinical Psychology* that "clinical psychology ... appears to have given little systematic study to the manner in which test findings are organized and formulated to provide necessary records and to render data easily and fully understood by professional associates" (p. 323). They expressed concern about the fact that "the many well-written, well thought-out psychological reports found in current practice appear to stem from individual institution or individual study of the problem of recording, rather than from a commonly accepted system" (p. 323). "It is conceivable," they argued, "that the psychiatrist or social worker who relies upon the work of the clinical psychologist may frequently be confused or frustrated because methods of reporting data are so varied and lacking in central philosophy and direction" (pp. 323–324). "Apart from [these] technical considerations," they further noted, "one's manner of relating to others and the way he feels and thinks will creep into his writing" (p. 332).

In 1989, **Reynolds and Mair** reported in the *Journal of Technical Writing and Communication* that "documentation in the mental health professions has received little study despite the fact that mental health records can be as crucial to a patient's well-being as medical records" (1989a, p. 245). They expressed concern that documentation standards varied widely, that they had found "only one point common among most mental health professionals working in the field" [their reliance on *DSM* nomenclature] (p. 246), and that "the factors that appear to have the most influence on document content are not immediately pertinent to patient well-being" (p. 253). "The communication situation is complicated," they observed, "by the wide variety of educational backgrounds of the various report writers and readers" who receive "little or no formal instruction in writing" and who instead "learn report writing during clinical practice, thereby learning from models—good and bad—and perpetuating the idiosyncrasies of reports at their host institutions" (p. 246).

The fact that these two studies, as well as most of those published during the 40-plus years in between them, so closely mirror one another raises some interesting preliminary questions. Why, for example, does nearly 50 years of professional work investigating the same basic research problem keep reaching the same basic conclusions? Why are key recommendations and conclusions (e.g., that mental health practioners need more training in writing and reading records) not acted upon? Is there widespread belief (and, if so, why?) that the difficulties associated with writing and reading mental health records are simply inherent and unsolvable? Are researchers addressing the problem of mental health records from so many different disciplinary perspectives that they are largely unaware of pertinent research published previously by researchers from other fields? We think the latter to be unlikely because at least some of the literature that follows crosses disciplinary lines, and either quotes from or makes reference to the body of work that

---

[1]Key researchers' names are in bold face at first reference throughout chapter 1 for readability and easy re-reference when we summarize patterns of research at the end of the chapter.

preceded it. In any event, we hope that the compilation and review that follows will prove especially useful to practitioners who must write and read these records daily, and to those who study the problem of mental health records in the future.

MAJOR CONTRIBUTIONS FROM THE 1950s AND 1960s

Sargent (1951) noted that written communication between psychologists and psychiatrists was "an important interprofessional problem," and that "the question of what a test report should communicate, and in what fashion, is a much discussed subject among both the writers and the consumers of test interpretations, but has not been answered to the full satisfaction of either" (p. 175). In order to demonstrate and compare different methods of reporting, Sargent presented four reports composed by the same psychologist about a single patient referred for acute anxiety and incipient schizophrenia. The reports, she concluded, differed in "purpose, vantage point, and logical orientation" (p. 184), and none "actually described the individual in a way which would make him recognizable among others except on close examination" (p. 185). Sargent concluded that the latter raised "a fundamental issue regarding the value of test findings" (p. 185), as well as the questions "What is the purpose of a psychological test report? Do we who write them share the purposes of those who read them? If not, who is to educate whom to their fullest usefulness?" (p. 186). Sargent argued for "greater flexibility and caution" (p. 186).

Foster (1951) reported that "most students in clinical psychology are poorly trained in report writing techniques." The cause, he felt, was that "their instructors, who, being psychologists themselves, accept technical test terminology as proper," and typically fail to focus on teaching their students how to provide information "in language which is meaningful in terms of the patient" (p. 195). Foster offered four simplified guidelines for better reports.

Lodge (1953) similarly offered beginning psychological report writers "a step-by-step guide [which they might use] until they have had sufficient opportunity to develop their own methods and standards for reporting" (p. 400).

Garfield, Heine, and Leventhal (1954) wrote of psychological report writing that "comparatively little discussion has appeared in the literature concerning this important activity," and that "critical evaluations of current report writing have been negligible" (p. 281). They distributed a 1-month sample of reports to all professional staff members in a mental hygiene clinic for their critical evaluation. Sixteen reports were analyzed and evaluated by 9 psychologists, 13 psychiatrists, and 11 psychiatric social workers. Noticeable differences between the three professional disciplines were observed. Psychiatrists, the researchers found, tended to be most critical of the reports, whereas social workers were least critical. The most frequent criticisms were that the reports were vague, unclear, speculative, inconsistent, and filled with technical jargon and clichés.

Cuadra and Albaugh (1956) prefaced their work by noting that "relatively little research has appeared which bears on the adequacy of psychological reporting *per se*," and that "no published research has dealt directly with the basic problem of communication" (p. 109). They presented four "representative, although not random[ly selected]" psychological reports to 56 "judges representing six professional groups" for their analysis and evaluation, and used questionnaires of both writers and readers to measure the degree of correspondence between the writers' intentions and the judges' interpretations. Results "indicated that communication was scarcely better than 50 per cent," and that "the greatest breakdown in communication occurred when the judges did not agree with the authors as to what was being emphasized" (p. 113). Caudra and Albaugh concluded that "there were relatively few *gross* errors in interpretation," and that "most of the breakdown involved problems in the specification of degree," but noted that "questions of degree are often of paramount clinical importance" (pp. 113–114). They recommended that report writers be taught to be "extremely explicit" and "direct" about their "points of emphasis" and "statements of degree" (p. 114).

Tallent and Reiss (1959a, 1959b) published a series of articles based on an extensive survey that "deliberately attempted to seek out the negative features of clinical reports with a view to publicize them so that they might be reduced in future writing." Printed research forms were mailed to 741 psychiatrists, 433 psychiatric social workers, and 393 psychologists, all of whom were employees of the Veterans Administration. Return rates were 81.2% for the psychiatrists, 97.2% for the social workers, and 97.7% for the psychologists. Respondents' criticisms were grouped as follows: problems of content, problems of interpretation, problems of attitude, and problems of communication. In analyzing their data, Tallent and Reiss reported finding "apparently meaningful patterns of criticism" showing "variations in preferences" (p. 446). Psychiatrists, for example, complained of too little raw data in the reports, whereas psychologists saw the reports as containing too much raw data. Psychiatrists wanted more direct reporting of patient behavior, whereas psychologists preferred more interpretation. Both complained about the absence of clear statements of purpose, and about excessive length, wordiness, and "deficiencies of terminology" (p. 445).

After noting that "amazingly little systematic attention has been paid to the writing of the psychological report," **Bellak** (1959) argued that the problems of communication in the mental health community "are variously inherent in the tools, concepts, and organization of the report itself." Furthermore, he warned, "Aside from the mechanics of the relationship, psychologists and psychiatrists are, of course, people. Their own emotions, value systems, apperceptive distortions, and their semantic problems enter into this area of communication" (pp. 76–77).

Feifel (1959) insisted that many of the "semantic obstacles" that interfere with written communication between psychiatrists and psychologists "stem from theoretical confusion" (p. 77), and suggested that communication might be improved if more research focused on clarifying the "frames of reference" and "working assumptions" from which the various practitioners' communications proceed.

Similarly, **Klopfer** (1959) described "the psychological report as a problem in interdisciplinary communication" (p. 86), and called for heightened attention to purpose, organization, and language. Klopfer advocated that writers determine their purpose on the basis of how their reader(s) would use their report; that they organize their work according to personality areas; and that technical terminology be "assiduously avoided." Further, Klopfer noted, "If the psychological report is to be utilized for a variety of purposes and is addressed to semi-professional and non-professional referrents as well as professional ones, it may be necessary to prepare several different reports. A report designed to serve too many different purposes [and, by implication, too many different readers]," he warned, "may serve none adequately" (p. 87). Klopfer recommended oral reporting as "the method of choice when communicating to school teachers, social workers, nurses, and other individuals whose professional training includes psychological matters only tangentially" (p. 87).

In 1964, supported in part by a grant from the National Institute of Mental Health, **Lacey and Ross** sought to replicate Tallent and Reiss' research, which had been conducted in Veterans Administration installations, in child guidance clinics. Their results suggested major differences between points of view in the two types of mental health care settings. Lacey and Ross attributed these differences to "structure, function, and interprofessional relations," and concluded that "a psychologist trained in a Veterans Administration setting will not readily find a child guidance clinic a congenial environment in which to work" unless he or she has had "specialized preparation not only in how to test or treat children but also in how to write acceptable psychological reports" (pp. 525–526).

Lacks, Horton, and Owen (1969) reported on their attempt to develop and subsequently test over a 6-month period a simple, standardized form for presenting psychological test findings. "In spite of the continued dissatisfaction with psychological reports throughout the years," they noted, "relatively little attempt has been made to actually change the form of these reports" (p. 386). They concluded that an outline form could be valuable in speeding up the writing of reports and also in presenting findings in a clearer, more concise fashion than the standard narrative form. They felt that the outline form would be particularly suitable in a setting that emphasized prompt evaluation over reporting extensive personality dynamics. The researchers also noted those studies that had preceded their own, commenting on the fact that "there seemed to be no consensus reached in these studies except that various professional groups in each setting differed on what they thought was desirable in a psychological report" (p. 383).

KEY DEVELOPMENTS DURING THE 1970s

The Problem-Oriented Record Movement/Debate

Grant and Maletzky (1972) were among the first researchers to note that well-kept patient records served multiple purposes in the mental health community. Records, they reminded their readers, had not only clinical but also research, teaching, and legal implications. Many patient records, they warned, failed to serve these purposes, because of "poorly operationalized constructs" as well as "purely mechanical reasons."

Given the multiple purposes that mental health records increasingly served, **Katz and Woolley** (1975) concluded that problem-oriented records (POR), as described and popularized by Weed (1968, 1969), offered promising improvements. "Problem-oriented records," they noted, "provide a potentially useful means of reorganizing existing patient records so that relevant clinical information is collected, displayed, and more easily dealt with in a logical way" (p. 123). The POR system (which advocated, essentially, that a patient record include an initial data base, a problem list, progress notes, and a discharge summary, and that the problem list provide the structural framework for all of the documents in the record) was seen by Katz and Woolley as having certain key advantages. First, problems are "functionally defined in behavioral rather than abstract, mentalistic, or diagnostic terms" (p. 123). Second, progress notes are "indexed by date, number, and title . . . and not fragmented by professional discipline" (p. 121). Third, discharge summaries "can aid in ongoing program evaluation, and be of considerable assistance to those who may be involved in the care of the patient elsewhere or on another occasion" (pp. 122–123). The basic principles of the POR format, Katz and Woolley contended, could be generalized to a variety of settings and treatment approaches.

Sturm (1987) reported that throughout the 1970s and early 1980s Weed's POR system was subsequently studied widely and debated in the mental health community. Sturm cited Biagi's work in social work, Haber's in psychiatric nursing, Miller's in clinical psychology, and Ryback's in psychiatry. "There have been many criticisms relevant to psychology of the value of the Weed system" (p. 157), Sturm noted. Of special significance to those interested in further exploring the POR movement of the 1970 is a study by **Webb et al.** (1980). It investigated the reliability of the POR system by examining the degree of interrater agreement among four therapists' ratings of the nature of the problem presented, and the severity of that problem, for 32 outpatients. Results indicated that the POR system was reliable for recording patients' problems on intake, but that interrater reliability for severity ratings was only 0.40.

The Siegel and Fischer Study

The most comprehensive study of psychiatric records to date, **Siegel and Fischer's** *Psychiatric Records in Mental Health Care* (1981), was the outgrowth of a 1974–1978 study conducted under the auspices of the Rockland Research Institute and funded by the National Institute of Mental Health (NIMH). The study consisted of three phases:

1. a review of guidelines for the content of mental health records as promulgated by various agencies such as the Joint Commission on the Accreditation of Hospitals (JCAH), state departments of mental health, and the federal government;
2. a nationwide questionnaire survey of more than 1,500 mental health professionals, exploring their uses of and attitudes toward records; and

3. an observational field study of record use within 18 varied psychiatric settings representing different treatment modalities and funding sources.

The book resulting from the Siegel and Fischer study was comprised of 14 chapters and spanned more than 300 pages. We believe many of its key findings apply not only to psychiatry, but also to the entire mental health community.

Chapters 1 through 3 focused on the uses, history, and contents of psychiatric records. The authors noted:

> The complexity of the mental health service delivery system has made the psychiatric record a multifarious document serving many roles. Its earliest historical utilization—as a teaching instrument—has given way to a great variety of other uses: clinical, administrative, accreditation, statistical, legal, quality assurance, program evaluation, research. How well the psychiatric record fulfills each of these roles varies and is highly debated. (p. 5)

From a purely clinical perspective, they added, psychiatric records are said to provide history, communication, and documentation; but the degree to which they are actually used in the clinical care of patients has never been fully determined. Additionally, the authors reported, "Despite the touted proclamations of the record's utility in administration, training and education, research, and program planning and evaluation, there was little available evidence to show that record utilization in these areas is widespread" (p. 9). Record-keeping in psychiatry, they wrote, has been most profoundly affected by three forces: the JCAH, Medicare/Medicaid and other third-party payors, and the *DSM*. In total, 17 separate sets of regulations governing psychiatric records could be obtained as of their study.

Chapter 4 presented details from Siegel and Fischer's national questionnaire surveying mental health professionals' attitudes toward psychiatric records. The 35-item questionnaire was mailed in April 1976 to slightly more than 4,000 practitioners. There were 1,557 final usable respondents: 529 nurses, 421 social workers, 322 psychiatrists, and 285 psychologists. Comparisons of the sample with national figures on staffing confirmed that the sample was representative, reflecting the national distribution of mental health occupations at the time. Highlights of results from the questionnaire included:

- The clinical parts of the records were the parts most frequently written and read.
- Psychiatrists were the highest enterers/writers of information, psychologists the lowest. Psychologists were also the lowest consulters/readers of information on the records. Nurses and psychiatrists emerged as the heavy record users.
- The survey found that 55.5% of the respondents kept their own personal records (i.e., they kept records other than those required by the care-delivery system).

- The two most pervasive problems reported by the respondents were illegible handwriting and too much information. The feeling that there were no problems at all ranked third. Ranking fourth and fifth were "missing information" and "disorganization."
- At least some relationship between good records and good care, according to 60.5%, while an additional 26% held that there was a strong relationship.
- Respondents in private practice gave "future use" as their second most common reason for keeping records; those working in state hospitals gave "communication."

Chapter 5 presented details from Siegel and Fischer's field study, which involved spot checks of randomly selected records, as well as interviews of clinicians. From September 1976 to June 1977, 18 clinical settings representative of state, private, federal, and mixed-funding facilities providing inpatient, partial hospitalization, or outpatient services were observed. Clinician record use was examined by means of a work-sampling technique in which clinicians were observed at 14 random time points during the day shift for 10 working days over a 2-week period, and then subsequently interviewed when they were employed in using a medical record or "at the time of other clinical activities with respect to their information usage" (p. 121). A final sample of 193 clinicians (40 psychiatrists, 40 rehabilitation therapists, 33 nurses, 31 social workers, 30 mental health workers, and 19 psychologists) provided 670 interviews. In each setting, 10 records were selected at random (180 total) and analyzed. Highlights of results from the field study included:

1. Treatment plans were missing from the sampled records about one third of the time.
2. Most records were in a structured (prompted lay-out) format; progress notes, however, were generally unstructured (no lay-out or inclusion prompts. Progress notes were also the part of the records most often recorded and consulted.).
3. Mean recording/writing time was 13.2 minutes; mean consulting/reading time was 9.2 minutes per record contact. Records were consulted mainly for specific information rather than general overview.
4. The information most frequently consulted was psychiatric findings, psychiatric assessments, and medication planning.
5. The records had varying relevance for the different disciplines. Psychiatrists, psychologists, and social workers consulted the record "to help make decisions." Other staff consulted the record "to get instructions."
6. Records for long-term inpatients were sparser than those of others. "These findings," the authors noted, "appear to support the widely held contention that less active treatment occurs in the care process for this population" (p. 130).
7. Respondents said they both entered and consulted treatment plans frequently; the observational field study did not find that to be true. "Treatment plans would appear in the record more often," the authors concluded, "if clinicians regarded them as useful and important, beyond merely fulfilling documentation of care requirements" (p. 131).

8. Respondents to the questionnaire said they most often entered data for clinical reasons and least often because they were required to. Respondents to the field-study interviews said they most often entered data because they were required to.

Chapters 6 through 14 of the Siegel and Fischer study presented essays contributed to the book by other writers who were specialists on issues of quality assurance, legal, training, and conversion to computerized records systems. Chapters 7 and 8, for example, offered two essays on accreditation issues; the first was contributed by McAnnich and Weedman of the JCAH, the second by Ozarin and Brands of the NIMH. McAnnich and Weedman wrote about the various monitoring and regulating bodies that reinforce the use of records for accountability purposes. "Accountability and documentation," they noted, "are the new games in town. Due to the increasing costs of mental health care, issues of third-party providers and political concerns relative to national health insurance, the professional clinician is having to become much more accountable than ever before" (pp. 230–231). In the essay that followed, Ozarin and Brands provided the useful information that "the single major reason for declaring a hospital out of compliance [with federal standards] is an inadequate or incomplete treatment plan" (p. 236). They also made two important recommendations. The first had to do with education: "Staff education about record-keeping," they wrote, "is essential, especially for newly hired staff. Many disciplines actively participate in the treatment process in psychiatric settings and write in the records. The education process must be hospital-wide and involve *all* treatment staff" (p. 241). Ozarin and Brands' second recommendation was for further research: "We are not at a point where we can say," they wrote, "that good records mean good treatment, though it is our impression that the two complement each other. More research is needed on the relationship" (p. 241).

AN EMERGING CONCERN IN THE 1980s:
THE WRITING OF CONSULTATIONS

Consultations in General

Commenting on the growth of consultation-liaison psychiatry, **Garrick and Stotland** (1982) offered a "detailed dissection of the anatomy of the consultation document to share [their] growing awareness of the profundity and complexity of the issues involved in writing a consultation" (p. 855). "The art and science of writing consultations," they noted, "has not been adequately addressed in the literature. Little has been published on the subject" and "from our own experience … we have developed an appreciation of the complex and profound issues involved in writing consultations" (p. 849). The authors reported finding the consultation's rhetorical context to be especially problematic: "The written consultation is meant to be read, for clinical and educational purposes, by many people and is available, for currently unavoidable reasons, to many others, who may read it for insurance or review purposes, out of idle curiosity, or even out of maliciousness" (p. 851). The "formulations" in consultative records, they especially warned, "pose the most delicate problems ... [in that] a human being with a constellation of complaints becomes a [label which is] poorly understood and anxiety provoking" (p. 853).

Consultations for the Courts

Hoffman (1986) reported that "the interface between psychiatry and law is very rough" (p. 169):

> There are a number of differences between consultation reports for another physician and those for a lawyer or court [in that] the psychiatric consultation to a lawyer is not primarily to influence the treatment of a patient but rather to describe and explain to the lawyer, the judge, or the jury the patient's symptoms and disability and their connection to a specific accident. The patient and others may have access to these medical–legal reports, and confidentiality cannot be assured. (p. 165)

Further, Hoffman noted that "the essential skills and organization for writing consultations are rarely taught during medical school or postgraduate training [and] many physicians have difficulty communicating medical knowledge to a nonmedical audience; this is especially true with written communications, which are neither stressed nor reinforced in medical school" (p. 164). Because psychiatrists are generally hesitant to get involved in personal injury cases and given no specialized training in how to deal with them, Hoffman further noted, "the bulk of the work falls on general psychiatrists [i.e., those who lack specialized training] or those who have shown special interest in the area [i.e., enjoy testifying as expert witnesses in personal injury cases]" (p. 164).

Williams, Dixen, Calhoun, and Mass (1982) reported that written records "function as the primary channel for communication between [practitioners] and decision makers (courts, parole boards, etc.) who utilize [report] information for determining sentences, treatments, types of parole, etc.," and that these records have problems of language, function, form, and confidentiality which have been ignored. "Studies evaluating the adequacy of psychological report writing have been sparse in the area of psychology in general," they argued, "and totally absent from the area of correctional research" (p. 126). "It should not be assumed," they warned,

> that correctional psychologists, probation officers and probation supervisors who regularly conduct psychological evaluations of criminal offenders have the necessary knowledge and skills to write psychological reports. In fact, the results of the present study suggest that a number of participants exhibited unacceptable and minimally acceptable report writing abilities. This finding is of great importance since improper and inadequate reporting of psychological evaluations results could lead to inappropriate decisions by judges who are responsible for the sentencing of convicted offenders. (p. 131)

Lanyon (1986) commented on other uses of mental health records used in court-related settings. The most widely studied aspect of the subject, he reported, is competency to stand trial, but the best known area of participation by mental health professionals in law-related work is assessments related to insanity defenses. These cases, Lanyon wrote, are especially difficult for writers:

> A common element of all legal definitions of insanity is that there must be a mental disorder. The mental disorder must bear a particular relation to the alleged offense. Add the further difficulty that the relevant period of time in question is during the alleged offense and not at the time of the insanity examination, and it can be appreciated what an awkward task such assessments are for the mental health professional. (p. 262)

Lanyon further analyzed writing tasks involving dangerousness, homicide, sex offense, and child custody cases; a mistake in the last case, he warned, can be "devastating" to the mental health of the children who "are often the greatest casualties" (p. 264) of the process.

Consultations in the Schools

Eberst and Genshaft (1984) reported that psychological consultations are frequently done for elementary schools trying to accomodate children with apparent learning disabilities, mental retardation, reading problems, behavior problems, and emotional difficulties. Recognizing the critical importance of consultative reports in such cases, Eberst and Genshaft conducted a study of the writers of psychological reports for schools. The study focused on examining differences between the report-writing skills of doctoral and nondoctoral school psychologists. Results indicated no significant differences.

Wiener (1985) studied the formats of psychological reports on children in elementary schools and how those formats might affect elementary teachers' comprehension of the diagnoses and recommendations being reported. Three formats were compared, and there was a highly significant difference between the three with regard to comprehension. Wiener recommended further research investigating format's effect on comprehension in secondary schools, special education centers, and other nonelementary settings.

Salvagno and Teglasi (1987) reported a study in which elementary school teachers rated the helpfulness of various types of consultative reports. No differences between test-based and observation-based reports, in terms of ratings for overall helpfulness, were found. However, the authors noted, the gender of the child being reported on did influence these "helpfulness" ratings; teachers rating the helpfulness of reports on males selected more recommendations for implementation than did teachers reading reports on females. "It may be that teachers are more concerned about the behavior of boys in the classroom," Salvagno and Teglasi noted, but "systematic research is needed on the impact of a child's gender and of style of report on the likelihood that recommendations will be implemented" (p. 422).

Wiener (1987) reported results from several follow-up studies prompted by her original 1985 study of elementary school teachers. Three studies of teachers' comprehension of psychological reports were described: a study of 42 school administrators, a study of 49 elementary school teachers, and a study of 77 secondary school teachers. Five report formats were compared, and it was found that "all three groups preferred reports in which both the child description and the recommendations were elaborated with explanations and examples and the structure of the report was highly salient" (p. 116). Wiener's results "contradict the opinions of many school psychologists who claim that teachers and principals 'do not read reports that are longer than two pages'" (p. 124), and this new "knowledge of readers of psychological reports needs to be considered when the report is being written" (p. 125). Written reports heavily influence decisions about placement and programs for children; thus, Wiener concluded, writers of psychoeducational reports have a special obligation to communicate with precision.

SUMMARY AND CONCLUSIONS

We began this chapter by identifying three themes that recur in the literature of mental health records, and in our review of individual articles we noted the themes most heavily emphasized in each. To further illustrate the recurrence of these themes in the literature, we would now offer the following lists of articles which explicitly or implicitly address each theme.

Theme 1: Relatively little systematic study of mental health records has been done, despite the role they play in patient care and management:

Taylor & Teicher, 1946   Sargent, 1951
Foster, 1951   Lodge, 1953
Garfield et al., 1954   Cuadra & Albaugh, 1956
Tallent & Reiss, 1959   Feifel, 1959
Klopfer, 1959   Lacey & Ross, 1964
Lacks et al., 1969   Grant & Maletzsky, 1972
Katz & Woolley, 1975   Webb et al., 1980
Siegel & Fischer, 1981   Garrick & Stotland, 1982
Williams et al., 1982   Hoffman, 1986
Eberst & Genshaft, 1984   Wiener, 1985
Lanyon, 1986   Wiener, 1987
Salvagno & Teglasi, 1987   Reynolds & Mair, 1989a

That 24 articles written over five decades all point to a lack of systematic study on this subject seems odd. We think this theme may recur as a result of several factors. First, rhetorical and linguistic issues in mental health records are generally outside the expertise of mental health professionals. Second, systematic study is made difficult by document cycles that vary from setting to setting and system to system, a subject we address in chapter 2. Third, many studies are done by academics, and universities are divided along disciplinary lines. The mental health profession, however, is multidisciplinary, involving psychiatrists, psychologists, nurses, social workers, occupational and recreational therapists, and others; and so research on patient records would require a multidisciplinary approach. Fourth, professional literature tends to be published and read along disciplinary lines. Some systematic studies have been published, such as Tallent and Reiss (1959) and Siegel and Fischer (1981); however, they were published in academic journals (which are particularly discipline-specific) or by presses that may not reach all mental health professionals. For these reasons, we think it is probably accurate to say that few systematic studies of records issues have been done, and that those that have been done may not be widely known across the professions.

Theme 2: Mental health practitioners receive surprisingly little training in how to write and read a record, given the amount of time they tend to spend doing both:

Taylor & Teicher, 1946	Sargent, 1951
Foster, 1951	Lodge, 1951
Cuadra & Albaugh, 1956	Hoffman, 1986
Eberst & Genshaft, 1984	Reynolds & Mair, 1989a

These eight articles, which explicitly or implicitly note the lack of training in writing and reading records in the education of mental health care professionals, cluster during the 1950s and then again during the 1980s. A remedy to this training problem would seem, at first, simple: Add a course on writing and reading records to mental health curricula, or address these issues in content courses already part of the curricula. However, implementing either is quite difficult. Curricular reform within institutions of higher education moves slowly, especially in areas of study with long traditions or particularly demanding programs with few electives. For instance, only in the last 20 years has technical writing become a fairly common requirement for engineers, even though the problem of "engineering English" has been a topic in the literature since 1893 (Mair & Radovich, 1987). Furthermore, instructors with training in writing and reading and an interest in the discourse of science and technology have been few and far between, and adding courses and faculty to teach them is an economic hardship in times of shrinking budgets for higher education. Training existing faculty to provide instruction in reading and writing is also an economic burden, and incorporating additional instruction into already full course plans is often seen as desirable but of secondary importance; in short, the inclusion of new instruction is seen as an academic burden. The difficulties of adding record-writing and record-reading instruction to existing curricula are numerous, but we must add our own voices to those of the authors just listed in a call for curricular reform. We also must applaud those instititions that have initiated their own in-house, inservice training programs to address records issues.

Theme 3: Communication among professionals in the mental health community is especially complicated as a result of its unusually wide variety of writer/reader backgrounds, care-delivery settings, and documentation standards:

Taylor & Teicher, 1946	Sargent, 1951
Garfield et al., 1954	Cuadra & Albaugh, 1956
Tallent & Reiss, 1959	Bellak, 1959
Feifel, 1959	Klopfer, 1959
Lacey & Ross, 1964	Katz & Woolley, 1975
Siegel & Fischer, 1981	Garrick & Stotland, 1981
Hoffman, 1986	Reynolds & Mair, 1989a

These authors cite one, two, or all three elements of this theme. A diversity of educational and experiential backgrounds is inherent to mental health care, but such diversity often causes problems for writers and readers, as the literature illustrates. Psychiatrists, psychologists, social workers, and recreational therapists speak different professional languages or, at least, widely different professional dialects; and even within professions there are different professional dialects/languages deriving from widely varying perspectives (cognitive-behavioral vs. psychodynamic vs. social-interpersonal, etc.). The kinds of interdisciplinary educational programs that might help develop common languages are not typical in higher education, and to expect the range that would be necessary to cover the many mental health disciplines would be unreasonable. An awareness of the varying backgrounds of readers by those writing reports, however, is not unreasonable, a subject we treat in detail in chapter 2. Differences in what individual records are called, the kinds of records (regardless of title) kept, and whether records are kept at all reflect the diversity of care-delivery settings, a subject also addressed in chapter 2. In a climate of govermmental deregulation, establishing a single set of documentation standards for all care-delivery settings seems highly unlikely and perhaps even impossible to do efficiently. However, these complications add to the difficulty of writing and reading patient records and need to be addressed.

A FINAL NOTE

We began this chapter by asking why nearly 50 years of research on the problems of writing and reading mental health records had not, apparently, led to the implementation of solutions to those problems. **Van Vort and Mattson** (1989) may have offered several useful answers to that question. They noted that although practitioners in the mental health professions are spending considerably more time these days on written work, "increasingly the record is perceived by clinicians as an accountability document rather than an important way to communicate with each other" (p. 407). The authors, themselves practicing psychiatrists as well as faculty members at UCLA and Cornell, wrote that inadequate training continued to present the single most significant barrier to improved written communication in the mental health community. Their own hospital, they noted, had begun conducting seminars, workshops, and lectures on writing, and "problems with documentation are now regular agenda items at our faculty meetings" (p. 408). (We would add two comments. First, there are multiple "accountability" forces at work here—malpractice fears, JCAH and other requirements, third-party payor needs, various reviews, etc.—and these forces are to some extent at odds with clinical functions; they deform and fragment mental health records. Second, "inadequate training" in written communication is not unique to the mental health professions; training in the use of the written word is, generally, inadequate in all of the professions.)

Van Vort and Mattson saw the second key barrier to problem solving as being *practitioner attitudes*. "Clinicians' attitudes toward and training in writing," they concluded,

> affect how well they cope with chart work. Writing can be a difficult, even onerous, activity, and clinicians who do not relish the task may find few incentives to devote time to it. Fulfilling documentation requirements limits the amount of time clinicians can spend with patients. Compared with the immediate reinforcement a clinician receives from regular verbal communication with peers, positive feedback for good written work is sporadic. In addition, the review of records by impersonal representatives of fiscal agencies rather than by clinical associates erodes confidence in writing as a valued professional activity. (p. 407)

Just as these attitudes toward writing present barriers to solving many of the problems of written communication in the mental health disciplines, so do certain attitudes toward clinical perspectives other than one's own. Apparently, there continue to be widespread and fundamentally inadequate understandings by caregivers of the important differences between the perspectives of the different mental health professions. Consultation between practitioners, **Bender** (1990) noted,

> requires greater communication efforts to overcome differences in respective areas of expertise and terminology. Collaboration is often achieved within institutions through multidisciplinary treatment planning and commonly accessed progress notes. The institution also provides practitioners with a geographic proximity that enhances interaction. Proximity and shared progress notes, however, will not necessarily ensure an effective team approach. Each discipline must also become familiar with the assessments and measures offered by the others and tailor their own activity to integrate with, and complement these other efforts. (pp. 18–19)

These problems and challenges offered by Van Vort and Mattson and Bender are formidable. In this book we certainly cannot solve and meet them all, but we have tried to make a beginning. We offer our analysis of issues associated with writing and reading mental health records in a nondiscipline-specific forum in order to raise important issues with and for all members of the multidisciplinary mental health community. We hope our work will make writers and readers of patient records more aware (and, perhaps, more wary) of the complex nature of the communication contexts in which records are written and read, and the attendant problems that derive from this complexity. We cannot offer recipes for writing perfect problem-free records; recipes work for cooking, but not for the difficult task of written communication about complex human behavior. Instead, we will try to frame and explore the major issues and then offer strategies that are flexible and, we think, valuable in confronting what are obviously difficult tasks. We hope that this review of the literature will help others who wish to study records issues in the future, that it will give them a springboard, a place to start.

Chapter 2

A Descriptive Taxonomy
of Mental Health Records

These initial contact notes—when they're actually written by a clinician instead of a secretary or a spouse—offer an interesting case study in what people from different training backgrounds perceive to be the important features of a cry for help, and they offer an outright amazing case study in how people determine the "appropriate practitioner" for a given client.

—Anonymous Community Mental Health Center Director

In 1986, having grown interested in patient records in the mental health professions, we decided to begin a study of the importance of written records in mental health care delivery by performing a rhetorical analysis of the documents typically written and read during the course of a patient's care. In order to perform our analysis, we had to begin by identifying the documents, and so we undertook the seemingly simple project of compiling a list, with descriptions, of the various documents involved in a typical patient care cycle. Somewhat naively, we assumed we could accomplish this first step by performing a single case study in which we would interview a mental health care team, collect samples of the documents that they wrote and read, and then analyze those documents. We found, and continue to find, that the situation is considerably more complex than we had expected.

THE MECHANISMS

Studying writing and reading in the mental health professions is complicated by two factors: First, there are many different mechanisms for delivering this particular type of health care; and, second, there are widely varying documentation requirements (in terms of both the records kept and the content of the records) for each mechanism. As shown in Fig. 2.1, our cases have now come to include five different mechanisms or settings in which a wide range of professional personnel deliver

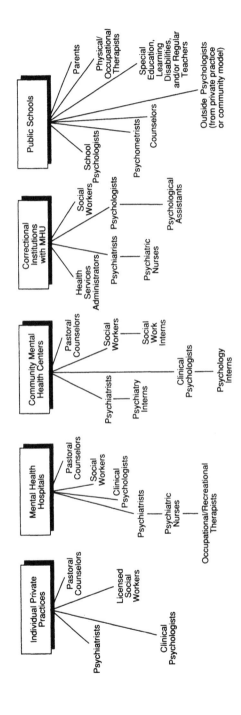

FIG. 2.1. Mental health care-delivery mechanisms and report writers and readers. There are five different mechanisms for delivering mental health care that we studied. Communication is complicated by the wide variety of educational backgrounds of report writers and readers.

mental health care. Originally we had thought there were three basic care-de-livery mechanisms, and we published an article describing them in detail (Reynolds & Mair, 1989a). As we continued to study mental health records, we added two more major care-delivery mechanisms to our list, and learned that there may be still more. For example, state mental hospitals and Veterans Administration (VA) hospitals, which we have just now begun to examine, may prove to be very different from the hospital/medical model we present here. Moreover, our interview data are increasingly indicating major variations between particular cases of each mechanism we have described. We have come to realize that our study will have to be ongoing, and that a complete coverage of all the possible variations may not ultimately be possible.

Individual professionals in private practice may not keep patient records at all unless third-party payors, fears of litigation, or other reasons prompt them to do so. Community mental health centers (i.e., the community model) typi-cally are subsidized nonprofit group practices that, by the terms of a contractual agreement with a subsidizing parent entity, are required to keep patient records. Mental health hospitals (i.e., the medical model) are public or private, profit or nonprofit, free-standing or specialized-unit entities that keep records in order to be accredited (e.g., by the JCAH), and to meet documentation requirements imposed by insurance companies and federal reimbursement programs. Correc-tional institutions, especially those with a mental health unit (MHU) on site (i.e., the correctional model) keep records in order to be accredited (e.g., by the American Correctional Association [ACA]). Public schools (i.e., the school model) differ from the others in that they do not provide care of the same breadth, depth, or, at times, kind as provided by the other models. We believe, however, that communication problems within the school model are similar to those occurring within the other models, and that the activities are at least related. Schools keep records because they are required by federal and state regulations to do so.

Within the community, medical, and correctional models, the communica-tion situation is complicated by the wide variety of educational backgrounds of the various writers and readers. Psychiatrists, psychiatric nurses, psychologists, social workers, pastoral counselors, and various types of therapists are typical writers and readers of patient records. During their educations, they receive little or no formal instruction in writing and reading records. They tend to learn report-writing during their clinical practica, thereby learning from models—both good and bad—and perpetuating the idiosyncracies of the reports at their host institutions. In private practice these problems are not as severe because records may not be kept at all, with the exception of reports for insurance companies, and if they are kept there may be only one writer and reader—cer-tainly there will be fewer and less diverse writers and readers than in the other three models. The school model is a middle ground in which the writers and readers may include school psychologists; outside psychologists; psy-chometrists; special education, learning disabilities, and regular teachers; coun-selors; and, of course, parents.

THE CASE STUDIES

One purpose of our study was to establish a descriptive taxonomy of the documents regularly written and read in the medical, community, correctional, and school models. We not only wanted to name these documents, but also to describe their rhetorical contexts. We wanted to determine each document's author(s), its purpose(s), its audience(s), and its use(s). In determining purpose(s), we were particularly interested in whether the primary aim was to persuade, to inform, or to instruct reader(s). (Because it was based on multiple case studies of a range of practitioners working in a range of care-delivery mechanisms, our work differed substantially from Siegel and Fischer's 1981 study, conducted from 1974 to 1978, which sought by questionnaire and field study to determine the types of information included in psychiatric records rather than the types of documents in which that information is contained. We think Siegel and Fischer's work is valuable reading for clinicians, and we refer to their work when calling attention to points particularly cogent to our own.)

In order to accomplish our goals, we interviewed the administrative head of a mental health hospital, the clinical directors of two community mental health centers (one of whom is also an adjunct professor of social work), the administrative head of an MHU within a correctional institution, a practicing psychiatrist, two practicing psychologists, two professors of psychology who specialize in mental health care in institutional settings, a pastoral counselor, a psychiatric nurse, two hospital records specialists, a record specialist within an MHU, four school psychologists, a psychometrist, and several special education and learning disabilities teachers. After determining that there were 5 basic documents involved (including one with 3 subdocuments) in the medical and community models, we collected 150 randomly selected sample documents written between 1982 and 1987. For the correctional model, we determined that there were 10 basic documents involved (11 in cases of commitment), and then collected 52 samples from five patients with complete files (two of the patients had been committed). For the school model, we were able to identify 4 basic documents, but were unable to collect samples. We combined information from our interviews with analyses of our 202 samples to determine the rhetorical contexts of the various documents.

THE TAXONOMY

As shown in Fig. 2.2, the care-delivery mechanism is an important determiner of both the number and the nature of the documents kept on any given mental health care patient.

As we indicated earlier, individual private practitioners may not keep records at all, and therefore are excluded from our analysis (which, we would remind our readers, is based on the settings we studied and may or may not be generalizable). In the medical model, 4 documents are typically written about a patient: an assessment (actually 3 documents reflecting three points of view), a set of progress notes, a treatment plan, and a discharge summary. In the community model, 5

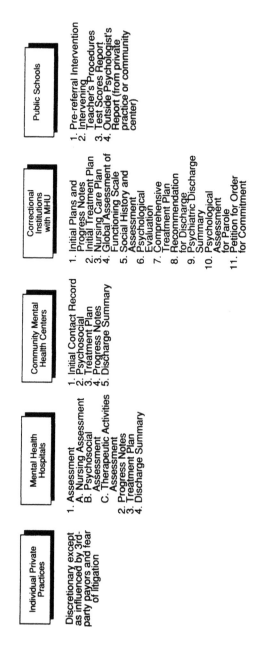

Individual Private Practices

Discretionary except as influenced by 3rd-party payors and fear of litigation

Mental Health Hospitals

1. Assessment
   A. Nursing Assessment
   B. PsychoSocial Assessment
   C. Therapeutic Activities Assessment
2. Progress Notes
3. Treatment Plan
4. Discharge Summary

Community Mental Health Centers

1. Initial Contact Record
2. Psychosocial
3. Treatment Plan
4. Progress Notes
5. Discharge Summary

Correctional Institutions with MHU

1. Initial Plans and Progress Notes
2. Initial Treatment Plan
3. Nursing Care Plan
4. Global Assessment of Functioning Scale
5. Social History and Assessment
6. Psychological Evaluation
7. Comprehensive Treatment Plan
8. Recommendation for Discharge
9. Psychiatric Discharge Summary
10. Psychological Assessment for Parole
11. Petition for Order for Commitment

Public Schools

1. Pre-referral Intervention
2. Intervening Teacher's Procedures
3. Test Scores Report
4. Outside Psychologist's Report (from private practice or community center)

FIG. 2.2. Mental health care-delivery mechanisms and documents generated. The care-delivery mechanism determines, in part, the number of records kept on a patient. There is obvious duplication of names assigned to records in the different settings, but there is little duplication otherwise.

documents are typically written about the patient: an initial contact record, a psychosocial, a treatment plan, a set of progress notes, and a discharge summary. In the correctional model, 10 documents are typically written about the patient who is discharged and eventually evaluated for parole: an initial plans and progress notes, an initial treatment plan, a nursing care plan, a global assessment functioning scale, a social history and assessment, a psychological evaluation, a comprehensive treatment plan, a recommendation for discharge, a psychiatric discharge summary, and a psychological assessment for parole. If the care team seeks commitment of a patient who is leaving the correctional institution, a petition for order for commitment is written. In the school model, 4 documents may be written to place a student in a special education or learning disabilities class: a pre-referral intervention, a description of the intervening teacher's procedures, a report on test scores, and an outside psychologist's report (usually from a psychologist working in private practice or a community mental health center).

Although there are some obvious similarities among names assigned to documents in the different settings, the variation is otherwise quite striking. In addition, beyond the obvious variation and diversity, a rhetorical analysis of the documents with similar names demonstrates just how dissimilar those documents are in these settings.

The Medical Model

Assessments. A *nursing* assessment is written by a registered psychiatric nurse within 24 hours of a patient's admission to a mental health hospital. Its purposes are to obtain complete information about the patient's physical, mental, and (sometimes) spiritual condition at admission, and to identify immediate problems and establish immediate goals and interventions. Because it is the first record generated, the nursing assessment is used to develop guidelines for the master treatment plan and, in effect, the patient's entire hospital stay. Any member of the treatment team may read the assessment. The team typically includes a physician, a registered nurse, a mental health technician, an occupational/recreational therapist, a social worker and, on adolescent units, a teacher and any assistants. The team may additionally include a psychologist, pastoral counselor, and/or another social worker who may (or may not) have been the referral source.

A *psychosocial* assessment is written by a staff social worker during the early part of the patient's hospitalization. Its purposes are to survey stress factors in the patient's environment that may contribute to mental illness, and to provide an alternative perspective to the nursing assessment (i.e., a nonmedical perspective). The psychosocial assessment is used to identify needs for social services. It may be read by physicians, nursing staff, and social service agencies (so long as the patient is hospitalized). If the patient signs a release, a copy of the psychosocial assessment is sent to the referral source after the patient is discharged from the hospital.

The *therapeutic activities* assessment is written by an occupational or recreational therapist. Its purposes are to determine the patient's leisure interests, and to identify problems associated with the patient's use of leisure time. This assessment is primarily used to create an occasion designed to promote the development of a personal relationship between the activities therapist and the patient. Any member of the treatment team previously indicated may read this document, and may use it as a guide for selecting interventions such as assertiveness groups, structured activities, or creative dramatics. The therapeutic activities assessment often concludes by identifying community resources that the patient might rely on after discharge from the hospital.

Progress Notes.   In the medical model, progress notes (and, almost always, admission notes) are written by psychiatrists and consulting physicians. The purpose of the notes are to document treatments given, to give rationales for medications and precautions, and to indicate continued stay criteria (such things as danger to self, others, and property; need for detoxification; incapacitating anxiety or depression; need for special medications or therapies; failure of outpatient care mechanisms). Progress notes may be read by all nursing staff, any member of the treatment team, the referral source, and any third-party payors. Nursing staff use progress notes to monitor medications and take recommended precautions. The treatment team and referral source use progress notes to monitor the patient's progress and to decide appropriate follow-up notations on the treatment plan. Third-party payors use progress notes to determine services that qualify for payment.

Treatment Plan.   In the medical model, the treatment plan is collaboratively written by the treatment team (ordinarily within 7 days of the patient's admission), with a registered nurse typically serving as recorder for the group. Each week, typically, the team then meets to evaluate the plan and update it. The purposes of original treatment plans (often called "masters") are to list reasons for hospitalization, to establish long- and short-term objectives, to characterize patient strengths and weaknesses, to specify time frames for care-delivery, to designate staff responsible for various treatments, and to reach consensus. The purpose of follow-up notations to the master is obviously to indicate changes, successes, and failures in the treatment plan. In the medical model, the treatment plan is thus used as both a document and an occasion to ensure coordination of care given by the multiple practitioners who comprise a patient's treatment team. We think it important to note that pieces from the nursing assessment, psychosocial assessment, therapeutic activities assessment, and (in the case of adolescent units) educational assessment are typically used to write the treatment plan, and that it is typically presented to the patient.

Discharge Summary.   In a mental health hospital, the discharge summary is written by a physician. Its purposes are to state the reason for hospitalization, to report any changes in mental status, to summarize medications given and procedures performed, to indicate any laboratory data, to state diagnoses at admission and at discharge, and to document any instructions given to a patient and his or her family about medications to be taken, stresses to be avoided, therapeutic activities to be continued, and so forth. Although it is not really its primary or, even, secondary purpose, the latter may be used to establish or preempt hospital liability in the event of litigation. The discharge summary may be read by social service agencies to which the patient has been referred, any insurance companies providing payments to the hospital and/or patient, and—in the not uncommon event of readmission—the psychiatric nurse writing the nursing assessment that begins the documentation cycle anew.

The Community Model

Initial Contact Record. An initial contact sheet/note records information from the initial telephone inquiry by a person (client or, often, family member) seeking services from a community mental health center. It is written, typically, by a staff person assigned to phone duty. Such duty is in most community mental health centers typically assigned to psychiatry/psychology/social work interns doing clinical practica in partial fulfillment of the requirements for post-bachelors' degrees. According to one of the sources we interviewed, initial contact records are commonly written by secretaries and receptionists, as well, unless center policies explicitly dictate otherwise. The purposes of an initial contact record are to gather information about the caller so that contact can continue, and to explore in a preliminary way the nature of the call so that the caller can be routed to the appropriate practitioner at the center. Initial contact records may be read by any inside/outside staff members who may have become involved in the client's treatment. These records are primarily used by the practitioner to whom the client is immediately routed, however, as an initial clinical assessment of sorts.

Psychosocial. In the community model, initial contact records take on further clinical significance insofar as traditional psychosocial assessments may not be written until a patient's fourth or fifth treatment session. (A center's contract with its subsidizing parent entity typically specifies some arbitrary deadline by which a psychosocial must be written.) The document can be written by a psychiatrist, a psychologist, a social worker, or a pastoral counselor—whoever proves to be the primary caregiver for the patient. (This may, of course, prove to be the practitioner to whom the patient was immediately routed, based on information contained in the initial contact record.) The purpose of the psychosocial in the community model is to provide a comprehensive written assessment of the client, based on personal and family histories and, often, interpretations of psychological tests of some kind. The document is used to establish possible sources/causes of the stressors that have motivated the client's appeal for help. The psychosocial may be read by any member of the center staff or treatment team and, with the authorization of the client, may be released to social service agencies.

Treatment Plan.   In the community model, the treatment plan is typically written by the primary caregiver. Its purpose is to outline the various interventions, therapies, treatments, and activities being recommended for the client. The document is used by consulting practitioners as the guide to be followed in delivering the services for which they have been assigned responsibility by the primary caregiver.

Progress Notes.   Any primary or consulting practitioner must append the treatment plan with a brief written record of any of his or her sessions with the client. These progress notes are primarily used by centers' subsidizing parent entities to verify that certain services were rendered. (Most community mental health centers have performance contracts with their subsidizing parent entities that, among other things, specify "units of service"—for example, "substance abuse counseling"—which the center must provide to the community during the term of the contract. Documentation audits typically examine progress notes in order to verify units of service rendered.)

Discharge Summary.   In the community model, the primary caregiver writes a discharge summary when the client terminates services at the center. The purposes of the document are to review and summarize initial diagnoses, all services performed at the center, and any resulting changes in mental status, and to document diagnoses/prognoses at discharge, as well as any recommendations made to clients and/or their families. The latter may be used to establish or preempt center liability in the event of litigation.

The Correctional Model

Before describing the documents for this model, we think it would be useful to describe a correctional setting with an MHU and explain why we chose such a setting for our case. An MHU is an on-site facility equipped to assess, diagnose, and deliver treatment to prisoners within a state correctional facility, and may receive referrals from other institutions within its state system. As of our first edition, the health administrator at our case study site believed that 6 other states had MHUs within their correctional systems, and she had received requests for information from 15 other states or U.S. territories that were either considering or in the process of establishing MHUs for their systems. In correctional settings that desire accreditation but do not have an MHU, the ACA requires that a mental health professional be available to perform initial assessments and refer those prisoners he or she thinks are in need of care to state mental hospitals with which the correctional institution has contracts for services. We chose a setting with an on-site MHU because of the growing interest and commitment to development of the MHU approach.

Initial Plans and Progress Notes.   A registered nurse is the first author of the initial plans and progress notes that begin with triage of the patient. The inmate (referred to here as "the patient," and also as "he" because the MHU serves the male prison population only) describes his complaint, and the nurse records it verbatim. The nurse then describes the history of the complaint, the patient's appearance, vital signs, the urgency of the complaint, and the immediate treatment, if any, and records whether the patient was referred to a physician's assistant, a doctor, or the psychiatric screening committee. If the patient is referred for mental health assessment, the purpose of the triage portion of this document is to provide the screening committee (consisting of a psychiatrist, a psychologist, and a psychiatric nurse) with basic patient information that is used to shape the screening interview. If the screening committee decides to admit the patient for mental health care, it describes further diagnostic plans, therapeutic plans and, when appropriate, educational plans. This portion of the document may be used by the psychiatric staff (the screening team plus the health service administrator, a psychological assistant, and a social worker) to write the initial treatment plans. The progress notes portion of this document is a chronological record with each entry divided into four sections: subjective (the patient's description of his condition), objective (usually the nurse's description but possibly any of the psychiatric staff's description of his condition), assessment (observer's evaluation of the patient), and plans (the observer's intervention). All members of the psychiatric staff read this record and do so regularly, but the progress notes portion is of particular use in writing a comprehensive treatment plan, recommendation for discharge, psychological assessment for parole, and psychological evaluation.

Initial Treatment Plan.   Typically within a few hours of admission (but not longer than 72 hours) the psychiatrist or senior psychiatric nurse writes the initial treatment plan. The purpose of this document is to record the patient's problems and the interventions to be used within the first 24 hours after the document is written. The description of problems is based on the patient's presenting problems, physical health, emotional status, and behavioral status; the interventions are used as instructions for nurses providing care during this initial period of treatment. Any member of the psychiatric staff may read this record. It is used most within the period of initial treatment, but the description of problems also is used in writing the comprehensive treatment plan. The ACA examines the document in evaluation procedures for accreditation.

Nursing Care Plan.   The psychiatric nurse writes a nursing plan for the patient within the first 24 hours after admission. The purpose of the document is to set goals for patient care and to provide instruction for the psychiatric staff and, in particular, nurses. Goals include a checklist form with entries such as "reduction of conflicts" and "improve grasp of reality," as well as space to construct goals. The document also assesses the patient and instructs by indicating precautions in checklist form with entries such as "aggression," "assaultive," and "suicide." Space under "other" is provided for additional precautions. The document also indicates whether socialization, self-esteem, verbalization, and responsibility should be promoted. Finally, the document records the problems and needs of the patient, and the approaches to solutions and the methods of evaluating them. Besides instructing nursing staff, this document is used by the psychiatric staff to write the comprehensive treatment plan. The ACA reviews the nursing care plan for accreditation purposes.

The Global Assessment of Functioning Scale (GAF).

The GAF is an assessment by a psychiatrist, psychologist, psychiatric nurse, or (sometimes) correctional officer of the patient's psychological, social, and occupational functioning on a scale of 10 to 90. The patient is assessed within 72 hours of admission and again at discharge. The purpose of this document is to indicate patient gains in previous care cycles if he is considered for readmission. The screening committee may use this document to shape the interview for readmission.

Social History and Assessment.

This document is written by the social worker within 72 hours of admission and is based on interviews with the patient and his family when possible. The purpose of the document is to acquaint other members of the psychiatric staff with the social background of the patient. It is written in narrative form and usually contains the following categories of information: early physical development, description of immediate family members and their interactions with the patient, description of schooling and social activities in that setting, hospitalizations for mental health care, sexual development, juvenile and adult court records, cultural and religious background, military and work histories, and drug and alcohol abuse background. The psychologist consults this document when selecting testing, and the psychiatric staff as a whole uses the social history and assessment in writing the comprehensive treatment plan.

Psychological Evaluation.

This document is written by the psychologist within 30 days of the patient's admission. It may be used in writing the comprehensive treatment plan, but more frequently it provides screening information for treatment teams at other institutions, or background for a second cycle of care within the MHU. The document contains a summary of presenting problems at admission, a history of admissions, a *DSM* axial diagnosis added at the time of discharge or transfer, behavior observations, psychological test results and interpretations, and conclusions and recommendations.

Comprehensive Treatment Plan.

This document is written collaboratively by the psychiatric staff, at times in consultation with a recreational therapist. Its purpose is to record consistently observed patient problems, set long-term goals and methods of treatment, and assess progress periodically. The document includes the reason for admission, a *DSM* axial diagnosis, presenting problems, treatment goals and methods, and progress. This document is reviewed if the patient's problems significantly change, and after the first 4 months of treatment in any case. The comprehensive treatment plan is used by the psychiatric staff as an overall guide for treatment and for long-term assessment of the patient's progress. It is also used to write the psychiatric discharge summary and is examined by the ACA for accreditation purposes.

Recommendation for Discharge.   This document, written by the treatment team (psychiatric staff, excluding the health services administrator and psychiatrist), records the ascent of all team members and a psychiatrist to the recommendation. The document also includes an inventory of completed reports. The recommendation is read and acted upon by the health services administrator, and is reviewed by ACA for accreditation.

Psychiatric Discharge Summary.   The psychiatrist writes this document to give an overall summary of a patient's stay in the unit when he is being transferred to another institution. It describes problems at admission, entering and exiting *DSM* axial diagnoses, GAF score at time of discharge, course of medication, discharge medications, and special concerns and recommendations regarding future patient care. Psychiatric staff at the institution to which the patient is being transferred use this report as background at admission screening.

Psychological Assessment for Parole.   The psychologist writes this report for parole board members, who seldom have training in mental health care. The purpose of the report is to describe the functioning and mental state of the patient while withholding any specific recommendation on parole. The report summarizes the patient's problems at admission, changes in behavior, relevant information from the patient's social history, and guidelines for continued treatment, if necessary, should the board decide to parole the patient.

Petition for Order for Commitment.   The court requires this document for involuntary commitment (even in noncorrectional settings). When the psychiatric staff believe that an inmate who has been a patient is a threat to self and society, and is about to be released from the correctional institution, the health services administrator may petition the court for commitment. The purpose of the petition is to persuade the court that the extreme measure of commitment is necessary. Typically the document outlines the number and duration of the patient's stays in the MHU and other state mental health care settings, describes current behaviors that are of concern, and includes an endorsement from the psychiatrist.

The School Model

Although we encountered variation from case to case within all models, no variation was so great as within the school model, where the documents varied as widely as the authors who wrote them. We would also note that the position within the document sequence that the report from an outside psychologist occupies can vary greatly from student to student within a single school.

Pre-Referral Intervention.   This document may be written by anyone who requests that the student be evaluated for placement, including parents, teachers, counselors, or principals. The purpose of this document is to identify students who may be in need of testing. The amount of information recorded (e.g., observed behaviors) varies widely. The school psychologist usually gathers additional information before deciding that testing is necessary and then requesting permission to test from parents. (Written permission to test is required by law, and in some schools the permission form asks parents to provide family, developmental, and educational histories. Those whom we interviewed told us, however, that this information is not required, that the response rate tends to be low, and that the best and most reliable information about histories is gained through oral discourse; we have therefore not included permission forms containing inquiries about history as a document in this model.)

Intervening Teacher's Procedures.   If the pre-referral intervention was written by a teacher, the school psychologist requests this description of class procedures used with the student over the previous 6 or more weeks. The purpose of this document is to provide the school psychologist with background that may allow him or her to develop classroom alternatives before initiating testing. If alternatives prove unproductive, the school psychologist will call a meeting with the teacher and parents and secure permission for testing.

Test Scores Report.   Testing and scores are provided by a psychometrist who reports scores and may or may not give a written interpretation of them. If no written interpretation is provided, the scores are explained to parents by the psychometrist, the school psychologist, a member of a regional special services team, or a school official. The purpose of the report is to help place the child appropriately.

Outside Psychologist's Report.   At some point in the placement process, the student may visit a licensed psychologist from outside the school (e.g., from a private practice or community mental health center). Parents may initiate this step or may be encouraged to do so if school psychologists and regional service personnel suspect the student may be emotionally disturbed. (Because staff members within the school model are not allowed to make diagnoses of emotional disorders, schools will often contract a licensed psychologist to diagnose these cases, or suggest that parents seek help from a psychologist of their choice outside the school system.) The outside psychologist will in many cases provide a report, but the nature of this report, which is to help place the student or to decide whether school testing should be done, can vary greatly. The most predictable element of the report is a *DSM* axial diagnosis (which is problematic because school psychologists, much less special education teachers or parents, are not trained in the use of the *DSM*). The document may also report results of various intelligence tests, projective and/or objective personality tests, apperception tests, and behavior observations. Interpretations and recommendations may or may not be included in the report.

SOME COMMENTS ON THE TAXONOMY

When we began our research, we were aware of neither the diversity of mental health care-delivery systems nor the impact of that diversity on patient records. We had envisioned codifying a simple pattern of documents, and then analyzing the rhetoric of those documents. Working from this perspective on pattern, we continued to find layers of complications until mounting data from an increasing number of cases (the number continues to increase as our research progresses) appeared to suggest chaos.

We then tried to shift our perspective on pattern away from its original narrowness and simplicity. We did not move to Siegel and Fischer's (1981) position (looking for patterns of information in documents rather than at documents themselves) because we were interested in the complexities and difficulties that mental health professionals face when reading and writing records, especially the very real problems that arise when records are transferred from one facility to another, within a model or across models. Instead, we looked for new and different perspectives on pattern that might emerge.

Variation of documents' names and, to a lesser degree, document inclusions emerged as one pattern. In all cases from all models we identified, those whom we interviewed commented on differences between records systems at their current and former job sites, or between theirs and colleagues' job sites. (Siegel and Fischer, 1981, focusing on kinds of information, could only identify "four *broad categories* of information contained in a record"; p. 25; italics added.)

Another pattern which emerged was the standardizing effects of outside forces. In each model, we found outside forces which affected documentation: accreditation agencies such as JCAH and ACA; federal agencies such as the U.S. DHHS; specific federal or state statutes, such as those governing educational opportunity; requirements of contracting parent entities. The specificity of requirements, the scope of the standardization, and the voluntary/mandatory nature of requirements, however, varied greatly.

When you work by performance contract, you agree to treat X number of cases of X different problems over X period of time. So frankly, then, when you get near the end of a contract, you do tend to start finding more cases of whatever you have left under the contract. Know what I mean?
                                               —Anonymous Community Mental Health Center Director

---

The wide variety of educational backgrounds of document writers and readers also emerged as a consistent pattern. In addition to the primary audiences indicated in the case studies just cited, we found that writers and readers of mental health records needed to be aware of additional secondary audiences. A draft version of the APA's *Record Keeping Guidelines* (1990) emphasizes the use of records by secondary audiences: "Users may seek psychological services for purposes of giving the results to others; they may need the information for third party payors or other sanctioners; and, the delivery of psychological services may subsequently become important for reasons unrelated to the initial request for psychological services" (pp. 2–3). Although various ethical codes and the laws of privileged communication protect patients from the disclosure of information given to clinicians, there are these exceptions: if the patient has given permission, if subpoenaed by the court or if the patient is undergoing court ordered treatment or psychological evaluation, if the clinician is a defendant in a lawsuit brought by the patient, if the patient threatens to harm him orherself or others, or if child abuse is disclosed. Although disclosure laws differ from state to state, it is generally accurate to say that anything written in a record may be disclosed in court if the court says so. This may explain why some clinicians said they kept notes that they did not put into their records.

A lot of my friends just keep two sets of records. A personal set recording what they really think, and an official set recording what they're supposed to think in order to get paid.

—Anonymous Psychiatrist in Private Practice

I don't think most people keep two sets of records, but I also don't believe that private practitioners keep no records at all. I just think they keep their unofficial records very, very private.

—Marcia Haynes, RNC, CHSA
Correctional Health Services Administrator

The special influence of the first document in a care cycle seemed to emerge as another, and perhaps the most major, pattern. That documents written early in a patient's treatment influence documents written later is not surprising. In some instances, however, we found that this influence may be disproportionate. As we noted in our discussion of the community model, the intake note may dramatically affect the mental health services the patient subsequently receives. As APA past-president Matarazzo (1990) observed, "the typical psychological examination carried out by the clinical psychologist is geared specifically to the benefit and needs of the particular patient, *determined from a careful reading of the patient's hospital chart, or in the case of an outpatient, from a telephone call or letter of referral*" (p. 1000; italics added).

In addition to these patterns, there emerged as a recurring theme the central and sometimes problematic role of the *DSM*. *DSM*-based axial diagnoses appeared in patient records in all of the models we found in our research. Perhaps the setting in which *DSM*-based documents seemed to be most problematic was the school model. Several school psychologists told us that behavioral recommendations are much more helpful to them than labels from the *DSM*, and that clinicians needed to write in language that teachers and parents can understand. Several studies have noted teachers' preferences for reports that consider these cautions (Salvagno & Teglasi, 1987; Wiener, 1987). The problematic role of the *DSM* in the other models is a more subtle issue that we explore in chapter 4.

Finally, we would once again emphasize that the specifics of our taxonomy, having been induced from individual cases, probably cannot be fully generalized. The consistent pattern of variation, diversity, complexity, and confusion that our taxonomy illustrates, however, appears to be representative of the overall system.

Chapter 3

Writer/Reader Biases and Mental Health Records

We are taught to make note of whether or not a client is well-groomed and presentable because this may reflect the ability to take care of oneself. But I suspect that comments about physical appearance (attractiveness, weight, style of dress, etc.) are far more often included in clinicians' notes about women than in clinicians' notes about men.

Does information about personal appearance tell us more about a woman than it does about a man? I suspect that this information goes in the notes because we are influenced more by how a woman looks than by how a man looks, and that it may seem relevant to us even when it has little or nothing to do with the woman's state of mental health or illness.

—Barbara A. Winstead, PhD
Clinical Psychologist and Professor

"The philosophical and theoretical beliefs of the psychological report writer," Hollis and Donn (1979) noted in their textbook on psychological report writing, "will affect the reports, whether this is done deliberately and consciously or fortuitously and unconsciously. Inevitably the writer's philosophy and theory will affect the terminology, the motivational emphasis, the conclusions, and the recommendations of the report" (p. 41). Everyone who writes and reads in the world of mental health will do so from a personal, philosophical, and theoretical frame of reference, Hollis and Dunn insisted, a frame of reference that includes "theories and beliefs about the nature of people, about the ways in which people develop and change, and about appropriate treatment programs, [and] naturally these beliefs will affect the interpretation and integration of data and information which in turn affects the reports one writes [and reads]" (p. 42).

Our research has led us to believe that Hollis and Dunn's brief introductory reference in this report-writing textbook to certain "writer/reader beliefs which affect interpretation" seriously underestimates and understates the complex nature and potential significance of writer/reader biases. Because we believe these important issues to have been largely unexplored in mental health records research to date, we want to examine in more detail the kinds of, sources of, and possible effects of writer/reader biases on mental health records. We want to affirm at the outset of this discussion that our use of the term *bias* is not meant to carry the common pejorative connotation of "unfounded prejudice." Instead, we use the word *bias* here in the sense of preference and/or predisposition, as a generic shorthand for the shaping of perspective on the basis of personal, philosophical, and theoretical frame of reference.

We use the term *bias* to denote what Welch (1987) called *ideological bias*, a shared system of belief, an interconnecting set of values that informs behaviors such as writing and reading. As Welch noted, ideological *bias* is "a largely concealed structure which informs and underlies our factual statements." It is "a system of belief which eventually becomes unconscious, making the objects of belief appear to be normal and natural," a kind of bias that over time "achieves the status of faith" (p. 271). (Or, as Vitanza, 1987, described it, the status of "common sense"; p. 85.) All of us who write and read, Welch insisted, are affected by ideological biases to which we have lost conscious access. "These deeply held beliefs present many difficulties," she explained, "because they derive so much power from their felt naturalness and normality" (p. 271).

The issues here—writers' and readers' beliefs, theories, values, philosophies— are, of course, quite complex. And the terms we must inevitably use in order to discuss them—words like *bias, ideology, fact, truth,* and *knowledge*—are, of course, powerful words, charged words, to some extent risky words. We believe, however, that discussing these issues in these terms is necessary and useful. Ideological biases affect our acts of writing and reading. Unaware of our unconscious predispositions, we write and read almost automatically. Accustomed to looking at our world from our own ideological vantage point, we come to think of language as "transparent" (Vitanza, 1987, p. 65) and underestimate the influence of the lenses and filters through which we see our world. In the discussion that follows, we look at the writing and reading of mental health records through our biased lenses and filters. We offer one way, an alternative way and we hope a useful way, of looking at mental health documentation. Throughout this discussion, we ask our clinician readers to temporarily step back from their perspectives and view their world from ours.

I am currently working with a child who has been to six psychologists this year, and each report has a completely different diagnosis.
—Anonymous School Psychologist

From our perspective, writers and readers of mental health records should consider these possibilities:

1. Mental health records are not only recorded information but also constructed interpretation;
2. Mental health records are communicative acts that are social as well as factual;

3. They are highly contextual, written within and for specific contexts, but often then read within and for others;
4. Not only the contents but also the language, focus, and form of mental health records reflect the biases of the professional communities for which and in which they are written and read; and
5. These communities are among the most complex in our society.

From our perspective, clinicians and others might use these alternative conceptualizations as strategies for achieving a fuller awareness of the complex relationship between writer/reader biases and mental health records.

THE SOCIAL CONSTRUCTION OF KNOWLEDGE IN PROFESSIONAL DISCOURSE COMMUNITIES

However a particular document from a given world of work is written, its reader(s) bring(s) to it a set of beliefs, values, requirements, and expectations as complex and elaborate as those of its writer(s) (Matalene, 1989). To the extent that these writer/reader beliefs, values, requirements, and expectations may be at least partially shared, the writers and readers in specific professional contexts belong to special groups or subcultures that writing specialists call *discourse communities.* Our world—a world of language—is made up of many different professional discourse communities, all of which use written language to "socially construct" knowledge. Inspired 20 years ago by Kuhn (1962/1970) and manifested in the work of Bruffee (1986) and others, "social constructionism" argues that knowledge, fact, truth, and reality are not absolutes but, rather, constructs generated by communities of like-minded or similarly minded peers.

Within the scientific community, for example, there is a fundamental like-mindedness about what constitutes "knowledge" and about the process required to construct it. Scientific knowledge is never constructed overnight but, rather, over time. Knowledge is rarely derived from conclusions based on a single experiment. Findings from single experiments achieve the status of knowledge only after being replicated by other researchers. Even after replication, findings and conclusions have still not become "fact" or "truth." Only after information has been disseminated to the community (usually by means of publication or conference presentation), and withstood the scrutiny of community members, do findings and conclusions become knowledge, truth, or fact. Scientific knowledge/truth/fact become so only through the process of communal assent, a kind of social construction-by-agreement.

Communal assent by the public then further validates scientific truth, especially psychological truth, a process that has been acknowledged and described in detail by Matarazzo (1990):

[T]here is no body of research that indicates that psychological assessment across the whole domain is valid or is other than clinical art. ... In this regard psychology is little different from engineering, medicine, or other professions. That is, professions in which practitioners' (artisans') work products are judged by society to be valid (usable) for many services, despite the absence of the necessary research, primarily on the basis that common experience (of legislators, professional peers, patients, clients, and others) suggests some utility from their services. ... [The] acceptance by these varied constituencies of a qualified practioner's work product as probably being valid comes only after a professional engineer, physician, psychologist, or other practitioner has (a) first met a set of educational requirements, (b) passed an examination and has become licensed or comparably accredited by the state, (c) had an in-depth review of samples of his or her professional work by members of a specialty board ofprofessional peers, (d) routinely shared and thus has had reviewed some of his or her clinical work products by peers who are also professionally involved with this client or patient, and (e) had those who have paid for and received such services conclude that the services were beneficial. (p. 1015)

The mental health community may well be the most complex scientific discourse community in which knowledge is socially constructed. The complexity derives from a number of factors, most notably the enormous diversity of practitioner backgrounds and care-delivery mechanisms, and can result in multiple levels of bias. Although we do not and cannot claim to analyze and illustrate all forms of writer/reader biases completely, we can analyze and illustrate several of them, and can offer two useful structures that writers and readers could use in conceptualizing the sources and manifestations of their own, and others', biases.

FOUR SOURCES OF WRITER/READER BIASES

Consider for a moment the primary writers and readers of mental health records—professional mental health clinicians. All are ideologically biased by at least four sets of influences. Figure 3.1 offers a graphic representation of how these sets of influences form layers of ideological lenses or filters through which writers write and readers read.

First, as human beings, professional clinicians unavoidably bring certain personal values and biases to everything they write and read. These values and biases derive from cultural and historical as well as biographical influences, because everyone who writes and reads does so from a particular point in space and time (Brower, 1959). Clinical assessment, Matarazzo (1990) acknowledged, is a "highly complex operation" that "rather than being totally objective ... involves a subjective component" that "cannot be separated from" the "values" (pp. 1000–1001) of the clinician.

Second, as highly educated scientists, professional clinicians add certain scientific biases to the equation. These biases, as we show later, affect both form and content because the scientific perspective involves beliefs not only about what can and cannot be thought of as knowledge, but also about how knowledge can (should) and cannot (should not) be expressed.

Third, as specific kinds of clinicians, professional mental health practitioners bring learned disciplinary biases to their work. Although educational stereotyping is not our aim here, it is nonetheless important to remember, at least in general

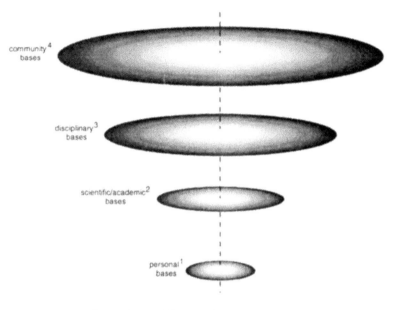

community[4]
bases

disciplinary[3]
bases

scientific/academic[2]
bases

personal[1]
bases

1 incl. cultural and historical influences
2 incl. notions about content, language, form, and focus
3 e.g., psychiatry vs. psychology vs. social work vs. pastoral counseling
4 e.g., hospital vs. community mental health center vs. correctional facility

FIG. 3.1. Layers of writer/reader bias.

terms, that there are key educational-background differences among professional clinicians: Psychiatrists are physicians trained to treat patients with multiple therapies, including psychotropic medications; psychologists are trained to provide psychotherapy and administer sophisticated psychological tests and assessments; social workers are trained to work with people within their social networks and environments; nurses are trained to monitor patient conditions, supervise care, and dispense medications; and pastoral counselors are trained to provide theologically informed psychodynamic psychotherapy (Schindler, Berren, Hannah, Beigel, & Santaigo, 1987; Young & Griffith, 1989).

Fourth, as specific kinds of practitioners working in certain kinds of group settings (e.g., hospitals, schools, mental health clinics, group practices, and correctional facilities), professional clinicians are likely to be affected by identifiable community biases when in the act of writing or reading.

FIVE MANIFESTATIONS OF WRITER/READER BIASES

Obviously, writer/reader biases can manifest themselves in a number of ways. A useful structure for grouping the ways in which writer/reader biases can manifest themselves can be derived from stasis theory, a classical system for dividing the analysis of an issue into five parts (Horner, 1988). Using the stasis system, we can identify five levels at which writer/reader biases might potentially manifest themselves in mental health records:

Level 1: FACT: What is it?
Level 2: DEFINITION: What is it called?
Level 3: QUALITY: What are its characteristics?
Level 4: CONSEQUENCE: What are its implications?
Level 5: POLICY: What should be done about it?

Consider, again, the primary writers and readers of mental health records—professional mental health clinicians. For them, all five manifestations of bias are possible.

First, professional clinicians writing and reading mental health records can be ideologically biased at the level of fact, which we use here in the sense of "event." Writers and readers can be biased about what is and is not possible, about what has and has not happened, about which behaviors are and are not identifiable as mental disorders.

Second, clinicians can be biased at the level of definition. Clearly, clinical writers and readers have learned ideological biases about what mental disorders can and cannot be called within their discourse communities. (It could even be argued that because clinical diagnosis is a form of rhetorical definition based on diagnostic criteria used in conjunction with a technical labeling system, mental health phenomena cannot really even exist at Level 1, at the level of fact. That is, it could be argued that a mental health event cannot really even occur until it has been named.)

Third, clinicians can be biased at the level of quality, ideologically predisposed toward certain beliefs about a disorder's severity, as well as about what are and are not a disorder's characteristics.

Fourth, at the level of consequence, the potential for clinical writer/reader bias is obvious. Clinical diagnosis will inevitably include professional value judgments about degrees of impairment, about what are and are not a disorder's potential consequences for a given patient.

At Level 5, the level of policy, clinical writers and readers can manifest learned discipline-specific biases about about what can and cannot be done, or about what should or should not have been done, to treat a given mental disorder.

These biases are largely unconscious and highly significant for the clinical writer or reader. Consider, for example, Level 1, bias of fact, bias about what has and has not happened, about what can and cannot be. Whether this bias derives from personal, scientific, disciplinary, or community influences, its consequences for the clinician writer/reader can be enormous. For any given practitioner writing or reading a clinical record, is chemical dependency a disease, a dysfunction, or a loss of self-control? Is incest a factual event, or a fantasy? Is hysteria an illness, or a form or resistance?

For the nonclinician writer/reader, bias at the level of fact can be even more influential. For any given teacher, guidance counselor, correctional officer, or parole board member reading a psychological assessment or other clinical record, what does or does not qualify as mental illness? According to Rosenthal (1990), many of the lay population believe "that there is no such thing as mental illness, just another way of looking at reality. That mental illness is a right to be exercised, rather than a disease demanding medical care." Similarly, a recent survey by the National Alliance for the Mentally Ill found that 71% of the respondents thought severe mental illness was only a display of emotional weakness; 35% thought it was not illness but a display of sinful behavior; and 45% believed that the mentally ill imagine their illnesses and could will them away if they wished. Forty-three percent believed mental illnesses are incurable, and only 10% thought that severe mental disorders had any kind of biological basis (Judd, 1990).

BIASES ABOUT SPECIFIC PROBLEMS
AND DISORDERS

Biases at the level of fact about mental illness in general can be exacerbated by fact-level biases about specific problems and disorders. Throughout the 1890s, for example, Freud himself wrote of a "frightening possibility" that kept emerging in his treatment of female hysterics. Each patient kept describing the same event in which incestuous advances were made by a father, brother, uncle, or cousin. Freud ultimately found it impossible to believe the women were telling the truth, and abandoned the notion of widespread events of incestuous advances as unthinkable. He found it "much, much easier to believe that every woman told the same lie, invented the same fantasy" (Carlton, 1990). Freud's rejection of the seduction theory in favor of the fantasy theory, according to Masson (1984) in *The Assault on Truth*, may have been "a turning away from the empirical reality, prompted by [his own bias], by [his own] general unwillingness to face the idea of sexual violence in the family" (p. 592).

Freud's personal unwillingness to believe in the possibility of widespread events of incestous advances appears to have been rooted in historical as well as biograph-ical influences. His own personal bias probably derived from a general unwilling-ness, rooted in late 19th-century thinking, to consider alternative perspectives on female hysteria. Throughout that historical period, Bledstein (1977) showed that gynecologists and psychiatrists regularly "diagnosed female hysteria as a patho-logical problem with a scientific etiology related to an individual's physical history rather than anger the public by suggesting that it was cultural problem related to dissatisfied females in the middle-class home" (p. 330).

Examples of fact-level biases about specific problems and disorders are not limited to the 19th century. They continue to manifest themselves in the scientific community today. In her study of the rhetoric of early medical reports on AIDS, for example, Reeves (1990) argued compellingly that preconsensus written at-tempts to diagnose and treat AIDS very clearly showed "groups in conflict want[ing] to make their interpretations the prevailing one of how things were and are and will be" (p. 394, citing Merton, 1973). The writers of the early records, Reeves concluded, "construct[ed] arguments with warrants that reached beyond the empirical data and called on premises about the nature of compelling medical mysteries," and made decisions based on bias, on "presuppositions, notions, and terms embedded in their interpretive networks" (pp. 397–398). In the mental health community, written attempts to diagnose, assess, and treat alcoholism, drug abuse, and PTSD—at least prior to their widespread acceptance as mental disorders—are likely to have manifested similar presuppositions, notions, and embedded terms.

(As an aside we would agree with Reeves, 1990, and argue that how the mental health disciplines establish and validate phenomena is an important question for both composition and mental health studies, and would suggest that preconsensus diagnostic records be studied in detail. For possible use in such research, Reeves suggested deploying sociologist Merton's useful distinction ,1987, between the cognitive and social patterns of "establishing a phenomenon" and "explaining a phenomenon." The former pattern aims at definitive characterization, whereas the latter pattern focuses on cause-and-effect relationships. Merton argued that unscientific and invalid discourse result from attempts to explain a phenomenon that has yet to be characterized or shown to exist. Mental health records attempting to explain certain phenomena before there was community consensus about their existence would be well worth studying in detail.)

BIASES ABOUT GENDER AND RACE

There is at least some evidence to suggest that clinicians may be biased at the level of definition on the basis of patient gender and race, that they may be ideologically predisposed to define mental illnesses differently for men than for women, as well as differently for Whites than for people of color.

The Report of the APA's National Task Force on Women and Depression (McGrath et al., 1990) cited "evidence that there may be systematic bias in the structure of diagnostic categories that results in an increased probability of misdiagnosis of depression in women" (p. 34). "For disorders such as depression that are congruent with gender role stereotypes," the report observed, "prevalence rates for women are markedly higher than for men. For disorders that are incongruent with society's idealized view of femininity and the 'good' woman (e.g., alcoholism is not congruent with idealized view), women's needs have been neglected and may go untreated" (p. 34).

I once read an admission note on a black client which said something like "Mr. X was very guarded during the interview. He gave very little information about his mother, and probably doesn't even know who his father is."

—Marcia Haynes, RNC, CHSA
Correctional Health Services Administrator

The report also cited evidence of the effect of patient gender and race on diagnosis even when clear diagnostic criteria are present:

Loring and Powell (1988) asked 290 psychiatrists to use *DSM–III* criteria to make clinical judgments with regard to the symptomatology demonstrated in two case studies that reflected actual cases receiving psychiatric treatment for undifferentiated schizophrenia with a dependent personality disorder. Indeed, that diagnosis was the modal response—38% of the psychiatrists applied it to the case. When the patient was described as a White man or when no gender or race information was provided, 56% of the psychiatrists chose undifferentiated schizophrenia as the diagnosis. However, when the patient was identified as either a Black woman, a White woman, or a Black man, the proportion of psychiatrists who diagnosed undifferentiated schizophrenia ranged from 21% to 23%. (McGrath et al., 1990, p. 34)

"Male psychiatrists were biased toward giving a diagnosis of recurrent depressive [dis]order to female patients," the report continued, [and]

were more likely to use the Axis II category of histrionic personality disorder when diagnosing White female patients, even though the cases used in the research provided little evidence for such a diagnosis. In contrast, regardless of their own race, female psychiatrists were more likely to diagnose White female patients as having a brief reactive psychosis. (McGrath et al., 1990, p. 35)

The results of the Loring and Powell study, the report observed,

are of concern to scientists who rely on clinical judgments in their research, as well as other individuals, including practitioners, who are concerned about proper treatment. Specifically, there is concern because psychotropic drugs used to treat depressive disorders are not the same as those used to treat undifferentiated schizophrenic disorder. (McGrath et al., 1990, p. 35)

BIASES ABOUT SCIENTIFIC
AND ACADEMIC DISCOURSE

The primary writers and readers of mental health records, professional clinicians, are in the larger sense scientists. But they are also highly educated academics. As scientific academics (hybrids), then, they tend to underestimate how heavily they are unconsciously influenced by conflicting biases about the natures of both scientific and academic discourse.

Generally, in their ideological notions about language and communication, scientists tend to be predisposed toward objectivity or foundationalism, toward what is sometimes called *logical positivism.* Scientists tend to be taught, and therefore tend to believe, that language is a transparent windowpane rather than a lens or a filter. Scientists tend to be taught, and tend to believe, that written communication can and should be faceless and passionless, that data and conclusions can and should stand bare and unadorned ("Just the facts, ma'am, just the facts"; Raymo, 1989, p. 26), that information can and should be evaluated for what it is, without prejudice or emotion or writer/reader reference.

Academics (admittedly not all, but certainly most) are generally taught, and generally tend to gravitate toward, a contrasting rhetorical bias, an unconscious ideological preference for seeing language and communication rhetorically. Academics tend to be taught, and therefore tend to believe, that written communication is analagous to oral communication, that speaker/writer and listener/reader are always as central to the act as is the message/text. Academics tend to be taught, and tend to believe, that discourse is always "talking" to someone, trying to have an impact on someone, and that most communicative difficulties and disputes and confusions come from assuming the "misguided" scientific bias—that discourse is detached, impersonal, and nonrhetorical (Elbow, 1991).

These contrasting and conflicting notions about language can dramatically affect professional writing/reading behaviors within the mental health community. Moreover, most mental health writers and readers are either unaware of, or unconscious of, the contrasting language biases pervading their educational backgrounds—and, therefore, their discourse community. As a result of these conflicting ideological stances on language itself, Masson (1984) noted, "Some analysts see psychoanalytic truth as an *objective, empirical* truth. Some analysts see psychoanalytic truth as a *subjective, narrative* truth whose standard is not correspondence with empirical fact but of coherence within discursive structure." (See, e.g., Donnelly, 1988, whose analyses and recommendations we confirm in chapter 6.)

In other words, some of the writers and readers of mental health records believe they are writing and reading truth, whereas others believe they are writing and reading interpretation. Some believe that in writing a record they are reporting a reality, whereas others believe they are constructing one. Some believe that in reading a record they are accessing a fact, whereas others believe they are accessing one version of it. Most, however, are unaware of these differences and the conflict between them.

Furthermore, for many readers, especially the nonclinical readers, Fish (1989) concluded that clinical case-history records, even when they are intended by their writers to be only versions of reality, tend to become reality. Removed from one person's context (and language biases) and read in another's, Fish argued, they "become installed at the center of a structure of conviction" where they "acquire the status of that which goes without saying, that which stands as irrefutable evidence of itself" (p. 547). (As Vitanza, 1987, would say, that which has acquired the status of "common sense"; p. 85.) In the discourse community of mental health, then, for clinicians and nonclinicians alike, writers who write, consciously or otherwise, from rhetorical/narrative/academic/relativist language biases are chronically undermined by readers who read, consciously or otherwise, from nonrhetorical/empirical/scientific/positivist languages bias, and, of course, vice versa.

OTHER KINDS OF BIASES ABOUT
SCIENTIFIC/ACADEMIC WRITING DONE IN GROUPS

As Matalene (1989) noted, writing often serves important functions for groups well beyond that of producing a document. Writing may have more to do with reaching consensus, setting goals, inventing solutions, revising priorities, or establishing control than the finished pages reveal. The records written and read in the mental health community serve important purposes other than the recording and communicating of information about patients, and those purposes lead to other kinds of bias in the writing done in the world of mental health.

As a number of the following scholars have shown, scientific and academic discourse are much more heavily predisposed than they realize toward certain kinds of language styles and patterns.

First, they are biased toward language that persuades. In many ways, the writers in a scientific/academic group seek not so much to inform their (or the other) group but to persuade it—to establish a phenomenon, support an argument, create a consensus, or even promote a conflict. Even the blandest reporting of information inherently must persuade the members of a group that the perception/view/description of reality being presented is a true one (Kinneavy, 1971). Similarly, even the blandest patient history must offer support for claims being made about the assessment of a patient or the effectiveness or ineffectiveness of some course of treatment (Reeves, 1990). With varying degrees of persuasive intent, professional writers always seek "to make their interpretations the prevailing ones of how things were and are and will be" (Merton, 1973, cited in Reeves, 1990).

Second, writers in scientific/academic groups prefer language that excludes ordinary people from their group (Elbow, 1991), language that validates the community's specialized training and unique insights.

They are also biased, according to Susan Sontag (1988), toward language that gains control of a problem as much as it explores and explains it. Particularly with "new" diseases, Sontag's research on the language of illness has suggested, writers are unconsciously concerned with "gaining rhetorical control over the illness," with gaining control over "how it is possessed, assimilated in argument and in clichè" (p. 94).

Perhaps because of their implicitly persuasive undercurrent, as well as their avoidance of exposure and liability, documents written by academics and scientists are generally biased toward language that communicates implicit rather than explicit themes (Reeves, 1990). They tend to employ language biased in favor of guarded stances and hedges, leading to writing that is at one extreme insecure, anxious, and defensive (especially of actions taken) and yet, at the other extreme, filled with elements of display which might sometimes be read as attempts to impress or show off (Elbow, 1991). (Naturally, we hope that the language of this book is positioned at neither of these extremes.)

The language of mental health is, generally, a language demonstrating a preference for narrative passive-voice constructions, a language that is inductive or indirect. And although passive/narrative constructions create the objective tone that scientific writers are trained to prefer, Reeves (1990) argued that "these bare, chronological orderings offer a subliminal appeal to emotion [with] parts arranged in order to make the greatest impact on the reader" (p. 406). Polanyi (1964) even argued that scientific writing's bias toward narrative unconsciously disguises the writer's selective inclusion and exclusion of information. "The quickest impression on the scientific world may be made not by publishing the whole truth and nothing but the truth," Polanyi insisted, "but rather by serving up an interesting and plausible story composed on parts of the truth" (p. 53, cited in Reeves, 1990). What is typically presented as induction, then, in scientific writing is actually deduction—the active imposition of regularities on the world, with much of the imposition, says Popper (1963, cited in Reeves, 1990), being a matter of guessing based on belief.

The primary way in which writers and readers in the mental health community "actively impose regularity on the world" can be found in their reliance on the language of the *DSM* as their primary vocabulary for written communication. This reliance, too, is a form of bias, an ideological commitment to the belief that an elaborate system of descriptive labels based on diagnostic criteria has been historically and continuously verified by empirical fact. (In chapter 4 we further discuss the ideological commitment to the *DSM* and suggest that its various revisions and refinements—even its current multi-axial diagnostic system—to some extent constitute efforts to reduce the effects of bias. However, as Robins and Helzer, 1986, observed, "While carefully defined criteria and explicit diagnostic algorithms clearly reduce the range of interpretation possible, no system is or ever can be so explicit than it cannot be bent to accomodate the diagnostician's own views"; p. 423.)

Grounds (1987) defended the mental health community's very bias toward the language of description itself, toward describing mental states in language that he said philosophers and laypersons chronically "misunderstand." "The conventional assumption that psychological reports [name and describe] inner states of affairs," Grounds insisted, is an "error" (p. 308). It is clearly not inconceivable to Grounds that descriptive psychopathology, the very notion of using written language to describe mental states, could be fundamentally biased or flawed.

ALTERNATIVELY DEFINING MENTAL HEALTH RECORDS

Writing and reading in the mental health professions, then, might be alternatively conceptualized as interpretive procedures (Carlton, 1990) climaxing in rhetorical definition (Elbow, 1991), the defining of mental health phenomena in context.

Mental health records might be alternatively conceived of as social constructions of truth (Fish, 1989) done in specific professional contexts (Matalene, 1989) for use by members of a complicated and elaborate interpretive network (Reeves, 1990) of both clinicians and nonclinicians.

Diagnosis might be thought of as an act of rhetorical labeling (disorder naming), based on reasons and evidence (diagnostic criteria), but also dependent on and filtered through a specialized and standardized vocabulary to which community members have ideologically committed over time (the language of the *DSM*), done by persons speaking with acknowledged interests to others—whose interests and positions one can ideally acknowledge and try to understand.

Mental health records might be recognized by both writers and readers, clinical and otherwise, as ideologically biased in a number of ways as a result of a variety of factors. They might even be thought of as to some extent recording and revealing as much about the biases of the writers as they record and reveal about the conditions of the patients.

Conceived of in that way, mental health records could be seen as much more than records. They could be seen as practitioner rhetorics and community rhetorics, communicative acts in which professional writers and readers define, redefine, confirm, and reconfirm their own beliefs and the beliefs of the communities in which they live and work.

Heightened writer/reader consciousness of these possibilities, we believe, would not undermine communication but enhance it. From our perspective, heightened writer/reader consciousness of records-as-rhetorics would lead to rethinking patient records as "histories not only of words but of silences," as records of what both has and has not been said, as records "infiltrated by [various kinds] of codings and decodings" (Carlton, 1990).

Heightened consciousness of writer/reader biases in mental health records might lead to "useful hesitations," to "prolonged moments of indecision" before making choices or writing things down; heightened consciousness might lead to writers and readers who pause before "assigning to a moment of discourse the status of truth" (Carlton, 1990). The aim here would not be to paralyze writers and readers of mental health records but, instead, to prompt them simply to hesitate. For clinician writers, the irony of such a prompt is not lost on us: We are suggesting that they hesitate at a time in which they are being increasingly pressured to include more and more information in their clinical records.

Chapter 4

More on the *DSM*: The Language System of Mental Health Records

It takes persistence to be a school psychologist, and a genuine desire to help a child. A school psychologist must spend an inordinate amount of time researching, interpreting, and translating the DSM terminology used in clinical reports for the various educational personnel involved with the child. What happens in schools that don't have a school psychologist? The information is useless to the school and the child.

—Anonymous School Psychologist

As we noted in earlier chapters, whatever their backgrounds, preferences, and personal or disciplinary biases, mental health professionals have one point in common. They all accept and rely on the language of the *DSM* for professional communication (if for no other reason than to secure third-party payment for services rendered). The first edition of this manual, *DSM–I*, was published in 1952. The most influential version, *DSM–III*, was published in 1980, and then again in a revised form, *DSM–III–R*, in 1987. A *DSM–IV* (whose "eating disorders" revisions were still being fine-tuned as our first edition went to press) was released in June 1994.

Each edition of the *DSM* has provided members of the mental health discourse community with a standardized list of mental disorders and their corresponding definitions and diagnostic criteria. (The more current editions of the manual have additionally prescribed a multi-axial classification system for the diagnostic assessment of patients.) Each edition has represented "an improvement over earlier versions" (McGrath et al., 1990, p. 33). However, as *DSM–III* and *DSM–III–R* came into wider use, "a number of issues were raised and continue to generate discussion and controversy" (p. 34). We believe all writers and readers of mental health records would benefit from a greater awareness of some of those issues, as well as a sense of the *DSM*'s history, its rhetorical limitations, and its pervasive influence on the mental health community.

54

We believe all writers and readers of mental health records, whether they be clinicians or nonclinicians, should understand this: The *DSM* language system—a technical vocabulary of descriptive labels with corresponding definitions based on specific diagnostic criteria—governs clinical diagnostics, assessments, evaluations, and recommendations (and therefore all written records) according to a system that was not originally designed for that purpose at all, but, rather, for national data collection (and which may have important limitations even at that).

I have to keep a medical book and DSM–III–R handy to decode these reports.
—Anonymous School Psychologist

SOME HISTORICAL BACKGROUND

The original edition of the *DSM* (*DSM–I,* 1952) attempted to standardize the nomenclature of mental health records so that national research data could be aggregated. *DSM–I* explicitly acknowledged this as its purpose, and in fact offered this important disclaimer:

> The general outlines above for the recording of diagnoses for statistical purposes, apply also to the recording of diagnoses on the clinical records. In view of the fact, however, that the clinical records fulfill wider function than the statistical records, the mere stating of the diagnosis (including its qualifying terms) is not sufficient for certain conditions, since it does not furnish enough information to describe the clinical picture. For example, a diagnosis "Anxiety reaction" does not convey whether the illness has occurred in a previously normal or previously neurotic personality. Furthermore, it does not indicate the degree and nature of the external stress nor does it reveal the extremely important information as to the degree to which the patient's functional capacity has been impaired by the psychiatric condition. Therefore, for most conditions a complementary evaluation must be entered into the clinical records. (pp. 46–47)

While edition *DSM–III–R* attempted to respond to the "growing recognition of the importance of having a common language for *both clinical practice and research*" (p. 1; italics added), several points should be noted. First, *DSM–II, III, III–R,* and *IV* will all reflect important changes, but they will remain revised editions of a manual originally designed for nonclinical purposes. Second, the influential third edition, by its own admission, "reflect[ed] [not a decreased but] an *increased commitment to reliance on data as the basis for understanding mental disorders*" (p. 1; italics added). Third, *DSM–III, III–R,* and *IV,* like their predecessors, were rich with disclaimers of their rhetorical sufficiency, several of which resonate with paradox. Important examples from *DSM–III* include:

- The manual names and labels several dozen mental disorders in 15 discrete categories after noting, "There is no assumption that each mental disorder is a discrete entity with sharp boundaries (discontinuity) between it and other mental disorders, as well as between it and No Mental Disorder" (p. 6).

- The manual implicitly acknowledges the risks of reductive labels by calling attention to a very fine linguistic distinction between its own, and other, phraseologies: "A common misconception is that a classification of mental disorders classifies individuals, when actually what are being classified are disorders that individuals have. For this reason, the text of DSM–III avoids the use of such phrases as 'a schizophrenic' or 'an alcoholic,' and instead uses the more accurate, but admittedly more wordy 'an individual with Schizophrenia' or 'an individual with Alcohol Dependence'" (p. 1).
- The manual promotes uniformity of clinical vocabulary but warns, "Another misconception is that all individuals described as having the same mental disorder are alike in all important ways. Although all the individuals decribed as having the same mental disorder show at least the defining features of the disorder, they may well differ in other important ways that may affect clinical management and outcome" (p. 1).

The *DSMs* thus have a history of which many writers and readers of mental health records are likely to be unaware. Each edition struggles to perfect what may conceivably be an inherently flawed language system not by replacing that system but by revising itself and then distancing itself, by disclaimers, from its predecessors.

I'll never forget that when I did my psych rotation, there was a list of acceptable diagnoses posted on the wall next to the charts. "Acceptable" meant that the diagnosis was listed in the DSM ... and that the insurance companies would pay.
                                                                     —Anonymous Family Practice Physician

---

Our purpose in calling attention to these distanced revisions and paradoxical disclaimers in the *DSMs* is not to blame but to warn. *DSM–III* itself urged caution:

> The purpose of *DSM–III* is to provide clear descriptions of diagnostic categories in order to enable clinicians and investigators to diagnose, communicate about, study, and treat various mental disorders. The use of this manual for non-clinical purposes, such as determination of legal responsibility, competency or insanity, or justification for third-party payment, must be critically examined in each instance within the appropriate institutional context. (p. 12)

We cannot help but wonder, however, how this caution is ever to be realized when these manuals govern all of the patient records written and read for precisely those purposes.

TWO FUNDAMENTAL WAYS THE *DSM* GOVERNS RECORDS

The more current editions of the *DSM*, as we noted earlier, prompt the form as well as the vocabulary of the records written and read in the mental health community. They do this by prescribing categories of, and numerical codes for, dozens of mental illnesses, and also by indicating that they should be presented in multi-axial format.

First, they present about 15 categories of disorders, each with subcategories, some with sub-subcategories, all with five-digit numerical codes. (The attempt, here, to facilitate future data collection, aggregation, and analysis seems fairly obvious.) The categories include:

1. Infant, childhood, or adolescent disorders (including nine subheadings such as mental retardation and attention deficit disorder, each with numerous sub-subheadings)
2. Organic mental disorders (including a variety of dementias as well as substance-induced mental disorders)
3. Substance abuse disorders (approximately 20, with "abuse" and "dependence" differentiated)
4. Schizophrenic disorders
5. Paranoid disorders
6. Psychotic disorders
7. Affective disorders
8. Anxiety disorders
9. Somatoform disorders
10. Dissociative disorders
11. Psychosexual disorders
12. Factitious disorders
13. Disorders of impulse control not elsewhere classified
14. Adjustment disorders
15. Other and additional disorders

Next, the manuals instruct clinicians to present their diagnostic evaluations according to a five-axes system. The first three axes constitute an official diagnostic assessment; Axes 4 and 5 are apparently not required, but simply recommended and available for use if desired:

Axis I: Clinical syndromes (the primary illness) plus additional syndromes (if more than one)
Axis II: Personality disorders
Axis III: Physical disorders and conditions
Axis IV: Severity of psychosocial stressors
Axis V: Highest level of adaptive functioning during the past year

(We would note here that there may well be an interesting correspondence between these five *DSM* axes and the five levels of potential writer/reader bias that we explored in chapter 3: the biases of fact, definition, quality, consequence, and policy.)

According to the manuals, "the principal diagnosis may be an Axis I or an Axis II diagnosis; but when the Axis II diagnosis is the principal diagnosis the notation should be followed by the phrase 'principal diagnosis'" (p. 24). Further, "when multiple diagnoses are made on a single axis, they are to be reported in order of focus of attention, [as in]

Axis I: 303.00 Alcohol intoxication
            295.32 Schizophrenia, paranoid, chronic" (p. 25).

A complete *DSM*-governed written diagnosis might therefore be presented as in the following examples (p. 30):

Example 1

Axis I: 296.23 Major depression, single episode, with melancholia
            303.93 Alcohol dependence, in remission
Axis II: 301.60 Dependent personality disorder
Axis III: Alcoholic cirrhosis of liver
Axis IV: Psychosocial stressors: anticipated retirement and change in resi-
            dence with loss of contact with friends
Axis IV: Highest level of adaptive functioning past year: 3—Good

Example 2

Axis I: 304.03 Heroin dependence, in remission
Axis II: 301.70 antisocial personality disorder (principal diagnosis); promi-
            nent paranoid traits
Axis III: None
Axis IV: Psychosocial stressors: No information
Axis V: Highest level of adaptive functioning past year: 5—Poor

The rest of the *DSM*, more than 500 pages long, presents diagnostic criteria describing each specific diagnosis that the *DSM* classifies and codes. Again, however, the *DSM* (somewhat paradoxically, we think) disclaims its sufficiency:

> These criteria are offered as useful guides for making the diagnosis, since it has been demonstrated that the use of such criteria enhances diagnostic agreement. It should be understood, however, that for most of the categories the criteria are based on clinical judgment, and have not yet been fully validated; with further experience and study, the criteria will, in many cases, undoubtedly be revised. (p. 31)

PROBLEMS WITH *DSM* SYSTEM VALIDATION

Writers and readers of mental health records, clinicians and nonclinicians alike, should be aware of some of the work that has explored questions about the reliability and validity of the *DSM* system. Of particular interest, we think, are (a) studies based on the NIMH's Epidemiologic Catchment Area (ECA) program, (b) a 1988 *DSM*-reliability study by Borus and others, and (c) a commentary by Matarazzo.

The ECA-Based Studies

The ECA program began with a survey interview study carried out from 1980 to 1984 in five communities in the United States by five university research teams in collaboration with the NIMH. The major goal of the project was to estimate population prevalence rates of selected mental disorders as defined by *DSM–III* criteria. By the time the first round of ECA-based studies began to appear in print in 1984, it had become obvious that the project had created opportunities for the research community to begin focusing on questions about *DSM* reliability and validity.

The ECA project included surveys of more than 18,000 household adults and 2,500 adults residing in institutional settings. Household face-to-face interviews were conducted with 18,572 residents of federal mental health catchment areas in New Haven, Connecticut; Baltimore, Maryland; St. Louis, Missouri; the Piedmont area of North Carolina; and Los Angeles, California. Interviews included the Diagnostic Interview Schedule (DIS), a highly structured interview created specifically for the ECA project for use by trained lay interviewers. The DIS contained questions designed to elicit the presence or absence of symptoms sufficient to establish the diagnosis of approximately 40 mental disorders according to computer algorithms constructed to general *DSM–III* diagnoses (Karno, Golding, Sorenson, & Burnam, 1988).

The ECA program was prompted by "gaps identified by the 1978 report of the President's Commission on Mental Health" (Regier, Myers, Kramer, Robins, & Blazer, 1984, p. 934), and by "an emerging NIMH consensus" that certain information was needed, including a test of "the utility of *DSM–III* diagnostic categories, as currently defined, to discriminate useful subgroups in both treated and untreated populations—in essence, a test of the *DSM–III* hypothesis that its operational criteria are useful discriminators" (p. 936). The ECA program has been called "a landmark in the development of the psychiatric knowledge base," and its data have been "extensively mined for a number of purposes" (Freedman, 1984, p. 931).

Data derived from NIMH's 1980–1984 ECA program have profoundly affected incidence studies, prevalence studies, care-utilization studies, and studies of targeted disorders for nearly a decade now, raising a set of important questions which we think users of the *DSM* might immediately ask themselves. Specifically, to what extent, if any, have ECA-based incidence and prevalence studies steered the diagnostic decisions of practitioners who have read them or studied them in school? To what extent have they constituted self-fulfilling prophecies; that is, to what extent do clinicians find what they have been led to believe they are statistically likely to find? McGrath and colleagues (1990), for example, cited studies that present "evidence that clinicians' beliefs about diagnostic base rates influence their diagnostic judgments" (p. 34).

In light of the enormous initial and continuing significance of the ECA program, we think users of the *DSM* should be made aware of the larger *DSM* validity and reliability questions that certain ECA-based studies gradually began to raise.

First, for example, some researchers observed that the DIS instrument itself had certain limitations. As Robins et al. (1984) noted, "The DIS did not attempt to assess all adult diagnoses within *DSM–III*. Even within those covered, some criteria were not assessed. Some criteria had to be omitted because *DSM–III* requires assessments that it was not thought possible for lay interviewers to make" (p. 950). Myers, Weissman, Tischler, Holzer, and Leaf (1984) further commented on the inclusions of the DIS and exclusions and explained how they were determined:

> Its selective coverage was determined through careful deliberations of a scientific advisory group, with decisions based primarily on expected prevalence, severity and clinical importance of the disturbances, research interest, and validity of the disorder category as suggsted by treatment response, family studies, and follow-up studies. (p. 960)

Second, some researchers realized that interpretive validity and reliability were ultimately dependent on DIS/*DSM* computer analysis. As Eaton, Holzer, Von Korff, Anthony, and Helzer (1984) explained, the DIS instrument "reduces information variance and response error to an absolute minimum" *because* "it also uses a diagnostic computer program to apply the rules for producing a diagnosis, which ensures absolute uniformity in the application of the diagnostic criteria" (p. 947).

Third, it was noted that certain *DSM* diagnostic categories are especially imprecise and dependent on human judgment and interpretation. Regier et al. (1984) acknowledged "the criterion variance inherent in some *DSM–III* diagnoses that are not sufficiently explicit to prevent multiple interpretations" (p. 940). Similarly, Robins and colleagues (1984) noted that "in areas in which *DSM–III* criteria were found to be ambiguous, the writing of applicable questions required making judgments as to probable intention" (p. 950).

One of the most revealing ECA-based studies (Boyd et al., 1984) "identified an operating assumption of *DSM–III* that has not received the kind of empirical research it deserves"—its exclusion criteria, its rules by which the presence of one disorder hierarchically excludes the diagnosis of another disorder when there are symptoms of both. The diagnostic criteria of *DSM–III* state that one diagnosis cannot be made if it is "due to" another disorder. Such exclusion criteria are found, according to Boyd and colleagues, in 60% of the disorders for which explicit criteria are found in *DSM–III*. The researchers found, however, using ECA data, "that if two disorders were related to each other according to the *DSM–III* exclusion criteria, then the presence of a dominant disorder greatly increased the odds of having the excluded disorder." Further, they argued,

> We also found that disorders which *DSM–III* says are related to each other were more strongly associated than disorders which *DSM–III* says are unrelated. However, we found there was general tendency toward co-occurrence, so that the presence of any disorder increased the odds of having almost any other disorder, even if *DSM–III* does not list it as a related disorder. (p. 983)

Most importantly for our purposes here, the Boyd study explicitly addressed some of the potential for *DSM* frailty that derives from written language itself:

The language of *DSM–III* makes a distinction between "essential features" and "associated features" of a disorder. For example, panic symptoms would be considered an "essential feature" of panic disorder, but an "associated feature" of major depression. This linguistic distinction, however, does not address the question of why panic symptoms occurring during an episode of major depression should be considered to be a manifestation of the major depression, and not a manifestation of true panic disorder occurring at the same time as major depression.

The use of the phrase "not due to" in *DSM–III* can be confusing since the phrase is not operationalized in *DSM–III*, and the definition of page 32 of *DSM–III*, does not indicate how one would determine if one disorder is "caused by" another disorder. Discussions within the ECA project have attempted to operationalize this phrase as meaning "not always occurring during an episode of." However, some ECA investigators take exception to this operationalized definition, since they interpret *DSM–III* differently. Some ECA investigators interpret *DSM–III* to mean that a disorder at one period of time might "cause" a disorder at another period of time, even if there is a symptom-free interval of many years in between. (p. 983)

The Boyd study ultimately found—and, we must stress, found great significance in—the "semantic confusions," "ambiguous phrases," and "linguistic distinctions" that lie at the very heart of the the dominant language of mental health, the language of the *DSM*.

In an overview for the first group of articles to appear from the ECA program, Regier and colleagues (1984) touched on the whole question of *DSM* validity and reliability while establishing the historical context of earlier epidemiologic studies. They described the Baltimore Morbidity Survey, a 1953–1954 project "designed to determine prevalence rates of specific disorders, levels of impairment, and needed treatment," and went on to say that "investigators used *DSM–I* as the basis for their diagnoses but made no attempt to assess the reliability or validity of their assessments" (p. 935). Regier and colleagues made several references to the validity and reliability of *DSM–III* and their relation to the ECA project, but tests of these were not identified as central or immediate objectives. The researchers noted, however, that "a useful data base will be available [from the project] to assess the validity of *DSM–III* diagnostic categories …" (p. 938). Near the end of their article, Regier and colleagues implied how this assessment might be accomplished: "The diagnostic criteria themselves are subject to predictive or construct validity comparisons with external criteria such as clinical course, genetic clustering, treatment response, and other characteristics described previously" (p. 940). The sense that validity and reliability of *DSM–III* needed to be assessed was clear in the article, but such testing was not an initial priority and still had not been undertaken as of 1986.

Two years after the publication of Regier and colleagues' 1984 article, the ECA program provided support for another article calling for assessments of the validity and reliability of *DSM–III*. Robins and Helzer (1986) traced the shift of the psychiatric community from anti- to prodiagnostic stances, and showed how this shift came to impact *DSM-III*. Washington University had long been a center (perhaps the center) for the prodiagnostic stance within the United States, and Robins and Helzer identified the "coincidence of Dr. Robert Spitzer's simultaneous roles as one of a small group assigned to define the areas of concern and diagnostic tools to be used in the NIMH Collaborative Depression Study and as head of the task force to produce the new official diagnostic manual *DSM-III*" (p. 413) as a very significant event in shaping the manual. While defining the areas of concern and the diagnostic tools for the depression study, Spitzer worked closely with and was influenced by Eli Robins of Washington University and his prodiagnostic stance. Spitzer was persuaded, through the collaboration and other events, that "atheoretical operational criteria for *DSM-III* would make possible uniform diagnostic practices even in the absence of shared etiological theories among the various psychiatric schools in the U.S." (p. 413). Many compromises occurred before publication, but *DSM-III* remains marked by this prodiagnostic influence.

What is of central concern here, we think, are some of the attendant conditions of this stance that Robins and Helzer (1986) pointed out, conditions of which many users of the manual are likely to be unaware. The authors noted that "the value of any diagnostic scheme can be tested empirically and that the current diagnostic scheme is only a set of hypotheses about reality, subject to change and development based on empirical research" (p. 414). In fact, the authors went on to quote Spitzer at length on this important question of diagnostic schemes: "Premature closure [of a diagnostic scheme] can be avoided only by the recognition that any classification system and its criteria should be regarded with *varying degrees of tentativeness* and should be subject to continued revision according to new knowledge. ... The specified criteria would facilitate rather than discourage future research because they would provide explicit definitions for the categories, *which would enable investigators to better study the comparative validity of alternative criteria* (p. 414; italics added). Robins and Helzer obviously shared Regier's concerns about the validity and reliability of the *DSM*. We wonder whether most users of the manual are as conscious of these untested aspects of their system.

Robins and Helzer (1986) described how *DSM* reliability might be measured using various structured interviews, including DIS:

> These multisystem interviews allow simultaneous assessment of multiple diagnostic systems in the same sample with the same interview format and the same interviewer, avoiding a number of possible confounders that would have to be taken into account if different instruments were used on successive occasions. By repeating this interview within a short time, the reliability of the [different diagnostic] systems can be compared. (p. 426)

The authors also addressed the issue of validity and how it could be assessed using the approach outlined by Regier, and by using structured interviews:

> The validity of a diagnosis can be assessed both in terms of its internal structure—i.e. its symptoms, response to treatment, and course—and in terms of its association with possible etiological factors. *At this stage in our understanding of most psychiatric*

disorders, validity cannot be ascertained in any absolute way. However, if a disorder has the same pattern of symptoms across cases and over time and is associated with known precursors, leads to predictable degrees of impairment if untreated, and responds to specific treatments, the chances that it is a valid diagnosis are greatly increased. The structured diagnostic interviews can serve for comparing the relative validity of the same diagnoses within the [*DSM*] system. (p. 427; italics added)

Prediction, Robins and Helzer (1986) thought, also could be used as a tool in validation:

When diagnoses are based on associations among features of the course and symptoms that are not themselves necessarily interdependent ... the chances that a true disorder exists is strong *just because there is no a priori reason to expect such correlations to exist.* These nontrivial correlations repeated in many individuals are an important form of prediction. ... Prediction outside of the symptoms of the disorder itself and their course is also valuable evidence for the validity of diagnosis. (pp. 428–429)

Our purpose here is certainly not to enter into an evaluation of the soundness of the authors' research design. Rather, it is to call attention to the ongoing concerns about *DSM* validity and reliability expressed by experts in the field, even by the head of the task force that prepared *DSM–III*. The ECA program provided a database that many think will allow for *DSM* validation and reliability assessments. As of the first edition of this book, however, no studies on these subjects were listed among the 247 publications collected in the "Publications of the NIMH Epidemiologic Catchment Area Program" available from NIMH. That such studies are needed seems apparent. Most important from our perspective here is that all users of the *DSM* should be aware of these needs.

The Borus Study

In addition to considering the rhetorical implications of the important *DSM* validity and reliability questions raised by Boyd et al., Regier et al., Robins and Helzer, and others, writers and readers of mental health records should also consider the implications of a 1988 study by Borus and colleagues. Their study was outside the ECA program, but it also focused on *DSM* reliability.

The study compared a group of primary health care providers' assessments of the current emotional disorders of patients just seen for an outpatient medical visit with those of mental health professionals assessing the same patients with the Structured Clinical Interview for *DSM–III–R* (SCID). (The SCID, like the DIS, is a structured clinical interview instrument designed to assess a broad range of Axis I and II disorders according to *DSM–III–R* criteria. The SCID was specifically developed to identify mental disorders often found in primary care medical practice.)

Using the SCID-derived diagnosis as the standard, the primary providers in the 1988 Borus study (internists and nurse practitioners) failed to recognize almost two-thirds of their patients with a current mental disorder. Although confident in their assessments, these primary providers were also able to correctly identify very few of the specific mental disorders most prevalent in primary medical care practice; they identified only one of the seven depressions, three of the eighteen anxiety disorders, and none of the four alcohol or drug abuse disorders. (p. 317)

More specifically, the primary providers in the study identified 22 of 88 patients (25%) as having a mental disorder, in contrast to mental health practitioners in the study, who identified 34 of those patients (39%) as having a mental disorder on the SCID. Only 12 of those 34 SCID-identified patients, however, were in the primary providers' group of 22; that is, the primary providers "falsely identified" 10 patients as having a mental disorder when they "did not have one according to the SCID standard" (p. 319).

Borus and colleagues concluded from their 1988 study that primary health care providers, "unfamiliar with the diagnostic criteria of *DSM–III* or *DSM–III–R*," do not recognize "most of the mental disorders their patients are experiencing" and, further, that the "providers' confidence in their evaluations is distressing" (p. 320). The Borus study thus concluded, essentially, that primary-care physicians do not reliably diagnose mental disorders. Although we are in no position to know whether the patients in the Borus study had mental disorders, we think it worth noting that Borus and colleagues did not appear to consider an alternative interpretive possibility: Mental health practitioners tend to find what they have been conditioned by their discipline-specific training to find, that their highly specialized language system—the language of the *DSM*—may work well for them, but not for everyone in health care. We believe, in other words, that Borus' study (and others like it) may further demonstrate our point about the mental health community's dependence on and committment to the language of the *DSM*.

The Matarazzo Overview

In a presidential address subsequently published in the *American Psychologist* (September 1990), Matarazzo provided what we believe to be an especially helpful summary and overview of what is currently known and unknown about the important issues of *DSM* validity and reliability. The following excerpts from that address speak, we think, for themselves:

> The portrait of an individual presented in such a typical 10–20 page report, whether accurate or not, is very different from the portrait communicated by a one- or two-word differential diagnosis, which is still too often requested by attorneys, insurance companies, and other third-party payors. In regard to the latter, many times during my nearly 40 years as a clinician-teacher providing clinical services to patients in a large university hospital, I have had to address the unreliability of such differential diagnoses offered by me or my psychologist and psychiatrist colleagues. In fact, because the published levels of clinician-to-clinician agreement were so low (*r*s of .20) for the diagnostic categories ... included in the earlier editions [I and II] of the *DSM* ... my colleagues and I carried out a federally funded research program ... in

an effort to help identify non-content parameters of the clinical interview that might help improve such levels of agreement across clinicians and thus help us better serve our patients. This research, begun in 1954, and my first literature review ... a decade later, of the research of other investigators, plus our own, continued to show that differential diagnoses such as depression, hysteria, and schizophrenia possessed little or no interclinician reliability. (p. 1012)

My subsequent review ... of research during the 1960's and 1970's ... indicated a considerable improvement. In fact, when I published my last review of this literature [in 1983] ... the levels of agreement in such differential diagnoses across two independent clinicians had improved materially. Specifically, for many of the discrete diagnostic categories in current use, the levels of interclinician agreement (i.e., *r*s above .80 and .90) now were being reported to be as high as the test–retest reliabilities of the WAIS–R and other well-standardized, objective tests. (p. 1012)

[I]t is my position that, after years of unacceptably low levels of agreement, the test–retest reliability of clinician-to-clinician diagnosis for a number of disorders has improved considerably during the past decade. (p. 1013)

Unfortunately, a widely publicized review of this same body of literature [Ziskin & Faust, 1988] reached exactly the opposite conclusion. (p. 1013)

My impression is that whereas 30 years ago almost *all* of the published studies relating to the degree of agreement on differential diagnosis of the disorders then listed in the *DSM* produced results that showed poor clinician-to-clinician reliability, my reading suggests that about 50% of the studies published in the past decade report good to very good magnitudes of reliability. (p. 1015)

Research that demonstrates the validity ... of such single- or two-word differential diagnoses, although available, is considerably more sparse for mental disorders ... although it is considerably more than adequate for mental retardation and the various gradations of intellectual ability. ... Therefore, in regard to the critical issue that the validity of *DSM–III*–type differential diagnoses has not been adequately established, Faust and Ziskin (1989) and I ... are in agreement. (p. 1015)

OF ADDITIONAL CONCERN: PROBLEMS WITH *DSM* NUMERICAL CODES

DSM-based mental health diagnoses involve the use of both words (labels) and numbers (codes). Most discussions, analyses, and critiques of the *DSM* language system have focused, however, only on problems associated with *DSM* words. Writers and readers of mental health records, we believe, also need to know about a significant problem associated with *DSM*'s numerical codes. Specifically, for example, the *DSM–III* system came into use in 1980, but many clinicians did not receive their new manuals for a considerable period of time and continued to use the old *DSM–II* system, apparently unaware of "marked disparities between the number coding of *DSM–II* and *DSM–III*" (Perr, 1984, pp. 418–419).

In a study published in the *American Journal of Psychiatry*, Perr (1984) reported several case studies illustrating the kinds of confusion and communication problems that resulted from the lack of numerical interchangeability of *DSM–II/DSM–*

III codings (and which we suspect may continue to result whenever *DSM* editions change). The following is one of Perr's illustrative case studies in its entirety:

> A major contest over a will hinged on the status of a patient, Mr. B, who had prepared the will while hospitalized and then died within 6 weeks after release. The major clinical issue dealt with the extent and fixity of an organic mental disorder. More specifically, the medical arguments dealt primarily with a differential diagnosis between delirium and dementia, and secondarily with the issue of symptomatic fluctuations and the possibility that Mr. B had had a "lucid interval."
>
> Three psychiatrists had seen Mr. B. Dr. A thought that the patient had an organic mental syndrome based on multiple physiological factors including cardiac disease, digitalis toxicity, generalized arteriosclerosis, and nephrosclerosis. He later categorized this condition as a delirium. Dr. B, in describing a similar clinical picture, made a diagnosis of psychosis with cerebral arteriosclerosis. Dr. C's findings were similar, stressing the deteriorating clinical picture over 6 months, the lack of recovery, and indications following study of the carotid artery of diffuse cerebral arterial disease with marked confusion, disorientation, and paranoid symptoms.
>
> Dr. B, in his formal report, made a diagnosis of "psychosis with cerebral arteriosclerosis, 293.0." To the consternation of the attorney who had employed Dr. B, it was pointed out that in *DSM–III*, 293.0 stands for "delirium," which by definition is generally transitory and of fluctuating degree. The differential diagnosis of delirium and dementia was crucial to the case; at stake was the disposition and management of millions of dollars. The matter was finally clarified when *DSM–II* was checked and it was discovered that 293.0 in that system was the code number for psychosis with cerebral arteriosclerosis. It was found that the evaluation, which had taken place in mid-1980, was indeed based on *DSM–II*. When Dr. B later received his *DSM–III*, he threw away his copy of *DSM–II* and then could not explain the apparent discrepancy until the differences between *DSM–II* and *DSM–III* were pointed out. Dr. B had clearly used the *DSM–II* wording and probably would have used the wording "multi-infarct dementia, 290.4," had *DSM–III* been in use. (p. 419)

This case, Perr noted and we agree,

> illustrates the fact that reliance on coding alone may create significant confusion, particularly when records from 1980 [the transition year between *DSM* editions] are reviewed. The fact that [a given coding number] stands for at times significantly different pathologies under *DSM–II* and *DSM–III* is an important matter to remember when reviews of case records are being done. Some conditions [26 of them] with different diagnoses depending on which *DSM* is used are listed in table 1. (p. 419)

Additionally, Perr concluded, suggesting some of the larger issues at stake,

> One might wonder about the accuracy of many statistical studies that use computer analysis, particularly when multiple, contradictory diagnostic systems are relied upon to various degrees and at different times in the course of one person's illness and when these systems have themselves changed every few years both in words and in symbolic representation of those words. (p. 420)

SOME FINAL THOUGHTS

As the 1984 Boyd study noted, any language system must serve the unrelated needs of different masters, and the language of the *DSM* must admittedly serve clinical, research, and accounting purposes. These purposes are inevitably, to some extent, going to be at odds with each other.

In a listing of six issues that challenge *DSM*, Robins and Helzer (1986) closed by emphasizing the problem of multiple users with different purposes: "Crosscutting these issues are questions about the competitive needs of researchers, clinicians, and administrators, who have differing requirements, particularly in terms of narrowness and precision" (p. 414). The authors continued:

> diagnostic systems serve many purposes, and it is unlikely that any one system [such as *DSM*] will be best for each of these purposes. They are used by administrators of hospitals, by departments of health for annual reports and budget requests, by doctors and patients making insurance claims, and ... as a tool for developing new knowledge about adequate treatment and about the nature of disorder itself. (p. 422)

We believe, all things considered, that the writers and readers of mental health records need to understand the dominant language system of their discourse community much more fully. We believe writers and readers would be empowered rather than restrained by better understanding their system's limitations and complexities. We believe that each *DSM*'s disclaimers are as important as its categories, codes, and diagnostic criteria. "Psychiatric research has been greatly advanced," one ECA research group commented, "by approaches to diagnostic assessment aimed at improving reliability" (Eaton et al., 1984, p. 947). Future studies should probably examine whether *clinical care* has been similarly advanced by DIS/*DSM*-dependent research.

Certainly, research and practice are as interdependent in the mental health community as they are in other professional discourse communities. In fact, because utilization studies are "used to provide estimates of the national requirements for mental health personnel and facilities and the costs for meeting the demand for mental health care" (Shapiro, Skinner, Kessler, Von Korff, & German, 1984, p. 972), they are probably even more interdependent. All of us, not merely the writers and readers of mental health records, would be better served by knowing that mental health policy, planning, and funding during our lifetimes will be largely dependent on ECA-data-dependent utilization studies of "specific mental disorders *as defined in terms of DIS/DSM–III*" (p. 971; italics added).

DIS/*DSM*-dependent studies have increased research interest in diagnosis, but Robins and Helzer (1986) identified additional factors:

> The interest in diagnosis that has captured the research community is being further stimulated by the tying of insurance company and government reimbursements to diagnostic decisions. We seem to have entered an era in which categorical diagnosis cannot be ignored because it will be the basis for deciding how many hospital days constitute appropriate treatment for a patient. Despite advances recently made in

studying course and treatability, this step seems a bit beyond what research data can currently support! (p. 43)

Exclamation points are seldom used in scientific writing, but we find Robins and Helzer's use of one here appropriate for calling attention to such a chilling prediction.

Chapter 5

Clinicians' Thoughts on Mental Health Records: A Pilot Survey

I used to work in one department of a large public hospital, a department which had been having so much trouble with Main Medical Records that it finally insisted on keeping its own records separately. Main Medical Records seemed almost always to be in a state of chaos. Employees chattering, radios blaring; staff (we can only hope) walking in and out, thumbing through the files, pulling some out and putting others back; no one apparently controlling or monitoring all the activity. Charts were habitually lost. Key information was chronically missing. Clearly the system was flawed. In fact, it was scary.

—Jennifer Ruhl
Former Hospital Data Services Specialist

In this chapter we describe the results from a short questionnaire survey of 47 mental health professionals in the spring of 1991. Our purpose in this pilot survey was to gather from a small sample of psychiatrists, psychologists, social workers, psychiatric nurses, and mental health counselors information about attitudes toward and uses of mental health records. We especially wanted to find out how much emphasis was placed on the importance of report-writing and record-keeping issues during educational and professional training programs, and to determine whether some of the concerns expressed by mental health professionals in the 1974–1978 Siegel and Fischer survey (published 1981) were still shared by those currently in the field. One primary purpose in conducting our pilot study, of course, was to determine whether the information derived from our questionaire survey made it valuable enough to replicate later on a larger empirical scale.

Our questionnaire consisted of 23 items grouped into two sections. The first set of questions gathered information about occupation, type of facility, years in the profession, theoretical orientation, and degree of emphasis placed on report-writing and record-keeping issues during professional training. Other questions in part one gathered information about the use of records in formulating diagnoses and treatments; these questions asked respondents to rank order the three most common difficulties with patient records, as well as the three most important functions that records should ideally serve.

The second part of our survey included a very short (and intentionally incomplete) hypothetical case. Respondents were asked to use their best intuitions and clinical judgments to diagnose the patient described in the case and to determine treatment modality, most appropriate setting and theoretical orientation, length of treatment, and diagnostic assessment procedures. Although we knew that the responses would not be true or complete indicators of the respondents' clinical judgments, we did think they would allow us to "get a feel for" the variety of ways patients are diagnosed and treated by care providers in the various mental health disciplines.

Although the significant limitations of our pilot study do not allow us to generalize beyond our sample, the results do suggest interesting questions warranting further study. The results support the premise that among providers there is a great deal of variation in the way patients' mental health problems are conceptualized and treated. The results also indicate that many of the difficulties with records that concerned the mental health professionals surveyed by Siegel and Fischer are still of concern two decades later.

The analysis of the survey data consisted of frequency counts of responses, and cross-tabulations of questionnaire variables. Small cell sizes precluded the use of nonparametric tests of the data.

DESCRIPTION OF THE SAMPLE

Respondents included 14 psychiatric nurses, 9 psychiatrists, 12 psychologists, 9 social workers, and 3 mental health professionals who classified themselves as "other." The majority of the respondents (40%) were employed in the psychiatric unit of a large teaching hospital, whereas 21% worked primarily in academic settings, 17% in mental health clinics, 11% in private practice, and the remaining 11% in "other" settings. Most of the respondents were experienced mental health professionals; 32% had worked in the profession between 11 and 20 years, 26% for more than 20 years, and 23% between 5 and 10 years. Only 19% had worked in the field for less than 5 years. The respondents identified their primary theoretical orientations as cognitive-behavioral (32%), eclectic (30%), psychodynamic (17%), family systems (15%), and "other" (4%).

THE EMPHASIS ON REPORT-WRITING AND RECORD-KEEPING ISSUES DURING PROFESSIONAL TRAINING

When asked how much emphasis had been given to report-writing and record-keeping issues during professional education and training, 47% of the respondents reported that these issues had received "a great deal of emphasis" during their training. When responses to this item were cross-tabulated with occupation, it became clear that psychiatric nurses reported this phenomenon much more often than did other professional groups. of the 14 nurses, 13 reported having "a great deal of" emphasis placed on the importance of records, with the remaining nurse-respondent reporting "some" emphasis. This confirms the findings of Siegel and Fischer, who also found that nurses reported a great deal of emphasis placed on the importance of records during training.

Of the psychiatrists, 33% reported "a great deal of" emphasis on the importance of report-writing and record- keeping during training, and 44% reported "some" emphasis. One psychiatrist (11%) reported "very little" emphasis being placed on writing during training, and the remaining psychiatrist (11%) reported "no" emphasis given to writing issues during training. Twenty-five percent of the psychologists in the sample reported "a great deal of" emphasis on records issues during training, with 50% reporting "some" emphasis. One psychologist (12%) reported "very little" training emphasis on records issues, and two (17%) reported "no" emphasis. One third of the social workers reported "a great deal of" emphasis on records issues in their training programs, and one third reported "some" emphasis. Twenty-two percent of this group reported "very little" emphasis, and 11% reported "no" emphasis at all.

THE RELIANCE ON RECORDS

Another finding similar to Siegel and Fischer's concerned professionals' views of the relationship between quality of care and quality of patient records. A majority (64%) of the sample believed that good care is at least "somewhat dependent" on good records, with an additional 26% reporting that quality care is "highly dependent" on the quality of records. Only 9% of those surveyed believed there was "no relationship at all" between quality of records and quality of care.

In determining treatment for a new patient, 45% of the sample reported finding previous mental health records "somewhat helpful," and 43% rated previous records "very helpful" in determining treatment. Eleven percent of the sample found records "only minimally helpful," and 2% reported that they did not refer to previous records at all in determining treatment.

Similarly, 62% of the sample reported that they relied at least "some" on previous records in formulating a diagnosis for new patient, with 15% reporting that they relied "a great deal" on previous records. Nineteen percent said that relied "very little" on previous records in formulating a diagnosis, and 4% reported that they did not rely on previous records in formulating diagnoses.

THE COMMON DIFFICULTIES WITH AND IDEAL
FUNCTIONS OF RECORDS

Respondents were asked to identify and rank-order the three most common difficulties with patient records, with a rank of 1 indicating the most common difficulty. "Illegible handwriting" (25%), "lack of information or missing information" (21%), and "takes too long to obtain records" (19%) were the difficulties identified most often by the respondents. Other common problems selected were "hard to find what I'm looking for" (12%), "records are too subjective" (10%), "information is not pertinent to my needs" (8%), "too much information" (5%), and "other" (1%).

When respondents were asked to identify and rank-order the three most important functions that patient records should ideally serve, with 1 indicating the most important function, the largest percentage (38%) selected "helping in the treatment of patients," 27% chose "communicating with other staff members," and 16% chose "having a written document in case legal problems arise." These findings mirror those of Siegel and Fischer, who found the same problems ranked in the same order.

I once worked with one doctor whose handwriting was so bad that after a few days had passed he couldn't read it himself and would constantly have to ask the nurses if they could tell him what he had written.

—Marcia Haynes, RNC, CHSA
Correctional Health Services Administrator

It appears that mental health care providers may keep personal notes about patients that do not become part of the permanent record. When asked if they wrote information on patients that did not become part of the record (such as scratch notes), 36% of the respondents indicated that they engaged in this practice "sometimes." An additional 21% responded that they did this "often." Twenty-eight percent said they "very rarely" kept personal notes on patients, and only 13% of the sample said they never did.

THE HYPOTHETICAL CASE

Respondents were given the following case and asked to respond to questions about it by using their best clinical judgments and intuitions:

Mary is a bright 12-year-old with her whole life ahead of her—except that she wants to die. Recently hospitalized after taking an overdose of aspirin, she has tried to kill herself twice before. At admission, she is diagnosed as severely depressed and appears to be making no significant improvement after 30 days of hospitalization. Additionally, she does not appear to be forming an alliance with her therapist and continues to have frequent suicidal ideation. Frustrated, her parents have discharged her from the hospital and brought her to you.

The largest percentage of the respondents (51%) recommended a combination of treatment modalities for the patient—individual and family, or individual, group, and family therapies. Treatments settings recommended for the patient were inpatient (38%), outpatient (34%), and partial hospitalization (26%). Two percent of those surveyed did not respond to this item. In terms of the most effective theoretical orientation to use with the patient, family therapy was chosen by 34% of the sample. Cognitive-behavioral therapy was selected by 26% of the group. Twenty-three percent chose psychodynamic as the most effective theoretical orientation for this patient, and 9% chose "other." When cross-tabulated with responses to questions about primary theoretical orientation, the reponses to this item were particularly interesting in their contradiction of any expectation that clinicians treat patients according to their own theoretical orientations.

Most respondents indicated that it would take at least 6 months to treat the patient in the case, with 34% recommending 6 to 12 months and 32% selecting 12 to 36 months as the probable length of treatment. Twenty-eight percent of the respondents chose 3 to 6 months as the estimated length of treatment, with only 4% selecting 1 to 3 months. One respondent did not answer the question.

Perhaps the most interesting finding was an apparent contradiction about the use of previous mental health records for diagnosis and assessment. Although the majority of the respondents (68%) indicated that they would rely at least moderately on previous records for diagnostic purposes, and an additional 11% held that they would make heavy use of previous records, only 19% reported that they would rely on testing results from previous assessment procedures in the case. Specifically, 62% of the sample indicated that upon being referred the patient in the case, who had previously been assessed and treated by other health care providers, they would retest with their own preferred instruments. Only 13% indicated that they would rely on results from previous tests administered by other mental health care providers. This would seem to suggest that much less credibility is given to test results than to other types of information contained in clinical records.

THE NEED FOR FURTHER STUDY

Our pilot study provided us with more questions than answers. For example, why did the respondents say that they would rely substantially on previous clinical records in the formulation of diagnosis and treatment for the patient in the hypothetical case, but also that they would give relatively little credibility to others' test results and interpretations in the patient's records? Since diagnostic procedures are quite costly in terms of both time and money to both patient and clinician, we are curious whether duplication is really necessary to ensure quality of care. Further study might help determine whether this practice derives from philosophical division in the mental health disciplines between those who believe in testing and those who do not, or whether it results from a more interdisciplinary debate driven by the reluctance to rely on results from testing over which one has no control.

Additionally, why (with the notable exception of psychiatric nurses) was there such inconsistency in the degree of emphasis placed on report-writing and record-keeping issues during education and training, even among professionals from the same discipline? This question is particularly interesting in light of the strict guidelines by which programs in psychiatry, psychology, and social work are governed and accredited.

The limitations of our pilot survey caution us against overly interpreting our data. After all, we know that a pilot study is just that. However, the results of our survey suggest that many of the problems with mental health records noted by Siegel and Fischer in the 1970s still exist, and that in an age of increasing accountability and liability for mental health professionals there are still many who get very little formal training, if any, in report-writing and record-keeping issues.

Chapter 6

Improving Mental Health Records: Instructional Strategies and Research Priorities

I used to think, as did many of my colleagues, that the increasingly litigious environment in which we worked had heightened our consciousness of the importance of what we wrote and how we wrote it. But I think the effect was largely limited to people working from the medical model, and I don't think the vast majority of us ever really knew what or how to do things differently than we were doing them.

—Robert C. Edwards, PhD
Retired Clinical Psychologist

During the four decades or so since the middle of the 20th century, the effectiveness of mental health care has improved dramatically. In his presidential address to the APA in 1990, Matarazzo personally attested to this dramatic progress:

> When I began my career in 1952, there were no effective treatments for any mental illnesses; it mattered little whether the diagnosis we gave a patient was schizophrenia, manic depression, or another disorder, inasmuch as the treatment (institutionalization) was essentially the same. For that reason, in hospital and clinic settings 40 years ago, even when a mistake was made, relatively little additional harm was done to those mentally ill patients. (p. 1001)

As modes of treatment became more numerous, diverse, and effective, however, both diagnoses and written records became more important. The latter moved from being short sets of notes and forms to being complicated collections of diverse documents describing, analyzing, and interpreting data and then translating them into complex diagnoses leading to treatments far more sophisticated than institutionalization. The evolution of mental health records was succinctly summarized by Soreff, Gulkin, and Pike (1990) in an article tracing the history of the patient chart: "In essence, the patient chart has gone from a simple collection of physician observations, reflections, comments, and recollections to a complex hospital medicolegal documentation system" (p. 127). As the authors implicitly indicated, litigation has affected the evolution of patient records perhaps as much as, if not more than, improvements in mental health care. And in addition to these two influences, of course, the part played by third-party payors has not been small.

One of my colleagues at the medical school once found himself in the unenviable position of having his records for one of the insurance companies being screened and evaluated by one of his first-year graduate students who just happened to be working for that insurance company part-time.
—Anonymous Clinical Psychologist and Professor

To some extent, today's mental health records still vary widely in length and complexity. Siegel and Fischer (1981) noted from their observations that "the content of an individual psychiatric record may vary from a minimal amount of information, such as the demographic data on the patient and the names of the treating clinicians, to tens or hundreds of typewritten pages in charts that have been prepared for analytically oriented case presentations" (p. 210). Our own experience in doing this research has been that today's typical mental health record usually falls toward the latter end of this continuum.

A widespread recognition of the growing importance of records issues in the mental health professions is evidenced by the APA's involvement. As of this book's first edition, the Committee on Professional Practice and Standards, a committee of the APA's Board of Professional Affairs, was in the process of revising a third draft of *Record Keeping Guidelines*, a document that will be the culmination of a project begun in 1988. The preparation of APA guidelines, however, is not the only indicator of the mental health community's concern about patient records; alternative approaches, some curious, are being offered. Proposals range from computer-based records systems (Barnett & Winickoff, 1990; Meredith & Bair, 1990) to systems in which "patients fill in their own medical charts" (Lanier, 1984, p. 189). In addition to proposals such as these, there have been calls for reducing diversity through standardization, a direction implicitly suggested by our study. We believe, however, that standardization would be problematic, to say the least. Siegel and Fischer (1981) agreed: "Obviously, not all facility types need the same data sets; an inpatient facility treating patients on a 24 hour basis requires different information from an outpatient facility seeing the patient for one hour every two weeks" (p. 211). Similarly, delivery settings other than those reflecting the medical and community models also have differing needs.

Although the mental health community has acknowledged the importance and problematic nature of writing and reading effective records, and has begun to explore solutions and improvements, much work remains to be done. In addressing mental health records issues, we see a dual approach as offering the most promise. First, instructional strategies, both immediate and long-range, could be implemented to improve the writing and reading of mental health records. Simultaneously, setting a research agenda for records issues, and then following through with that agenda, could both shape long-range strategies and measure the effectiveness of immediate strategies. A dual approach would allow a reciprocity between research and instruction. The ultimate goal would be to understand how records influence care, and to discover how records can be reshaped to improve care.

INSTRUCTIONAL STRATEGIES

Some of the instructional strategies that can be implemented immediately are quite simple. For example, teaching "complete documentation" would seem rather mechanical, but considering the fact that the *DSM* has already gone through five editions (*DSM–I* through *DSM–III–R* plus *DSM–IV*), complete documentation becomes an absolute imperative. As Perr (1984) warned, "number alone without information as to time, manual used, context, or adequate verbal description can result in erroneous interpretation. In everyday work it might be advantageous to spell out the reference methodology (e.g., *DSM–III*, 293.0, rather than just 293.0)" (p. 419), since the resulting confusions have serious consequences. Teaching current and future clinicians the simple solution to this particular problem would be easy.

An example of a somewhat less mechanical and yet still easily implemented instructional strategy would be teaching writers to identify clearly and explicitly the purpose, audience, and use of a document, and conclusions that are tentative as such. Having demonstrated the diversity of readership for mental health records, we believe the explicit identification of a document's intended purpose, audience, and use would reduce the chance of it being unknowingly interpreted inappropriately in another rhetorical context. This strategy of explicit identification could also be applied to conclusions. As the third draft of the APA's *Record Keeping Guidelines* (1990) states, "Psychological services routinely involve inferences that are subjective, tentative, or subject to substantial revisions based on further work. *The tentative nature of such inferences should be recorded*" (p. 8; italics added).

In addition to these concrete instructional strategies that could be implemented immediately, we believe long-range strategies for dealing with the more abstract conceptual records issues need to be developed and implemented in the near future. Fundamental conceptions of mental health records need to be reevaluated so that writers and readers can become more self-conscious. As Donnelly (1988) noted, for example, physicians need to learn that patient histories are "not taken, but made," that they are "created, not found. Furthermore, whatever we physicians compose and record as history is not "reality" in any global sense, but one version of reality, one that we choose to construct" (p. 824). If writers and readers of mental health records were taught this concept as a whole, then individual documents within a patient record would come to be viewed in the same way. As Hollis and Donn (1979) observed, writers and readers must be alert to limitations of using earlier reports as a source of data and information. Earlier reports or documents might have been written for different purposes and different readers from those intended by the current report writer. In addition, another hazard is the possibility that earlier reports or documents might serve to bias the current writer. (p. 33)

Only by conceiving of earlier reports as one construction of reality can writers and readers engage in useful hesitations that avoid the disproportionate influences of these documents.

Because we believe that both immediate and long-range instructional strategies can be used to improve the written records that facilitate mental health care, we remain convinced that curricular reform—despite its difficulty and expense—is a necessary and potent variable in the mental health care equation. Formal instruction in writing and reading mental health records must be incorporated into the graduate and continuing educations of mental health care professionals. We envision this instruction as raising the widest possible range of writing/reading issues, thereby heightening the consciousness of future clinicians. Complex, realistic cases centering on patient records could be used during instruction to simulate the kinds of challenges students will face as professionals. These cases could offer opportunities for role-playing and discussion of difficult writing/reading issues. Instruction could be carried on by multidisciplinary teams, helping students experience firsthand a diversity of audiences and document uses.

The multidisciplinary approach in the educational setting could strategically be extended to the professional setting. Communication among members of the various mental health disciplines and those working in the various care-delivery settings would promote a heightened professional self-consciousness. If publication boundaries between disciplines are so rigid as to make communication difficult or impossible, then professional organizations should consider making time available at their conferences for speakers who represent areas allied to, but other than, their own. Another strategy here would be conferences that are jointly sponsored by different professional organizations and that address issues and problems arising from the diversity of readers and uses of records. This approach could be extended further by communication among the appropriate subcommittees of the various accrediting agencies that address issues associated with mental health records.

RESEARCH PRIORITIES

While immediate instructional strategies are being implemented and long-range strategies are being developed and refined, qualitative research can discover and identify important records questions and perhaps suggest directions in which answers might profitably be sought. Knowledge gained from this research could then be used to guide the development of additional instructional strategies whose effectiveness could then be tested through additional research.

We think that additional case studies of the models we have identified (and perhaps others we have not included) might provide a clearer sense of the extent of the current variation and diversity, and perhaps reveal patterns we did not

perceive. This research might suggest directions for quantitative descriptive research. Case studies utilizing think-aloud protocols of writers and readers of mental
health records might also be valuable in generating hypotheses to be tested in other
designs. Long-term studies similar to ethnographies also might yield data about
records within various delivery settings and help us generate hypotheses.

Studies of the impact of document design (organization and format) might reveal
information about the relative effectiveness or efficiency of various record lay-out
patterns. Once the validity and reliability of *DSM*-based diagnoses have been
determined, the question of how these diagnoses affect the wide range of patient-
record readers remains to be explored, as well as the question (even in the most
relative sense) of how early documents impact the reading and writing of documents positioned later in care-delivery sequences. External factors such as the
influence of third-party payors are numerous and difficult; they may prove impossible to measure.

The research agenda is already long. In all likelihood, it will grow longer. We
realize that qualitative research in this realm, let alone quantitative research, will
be difficult. We remain convinced, however, that the growing concern about records
indicates the mental health community's willingness to tackle this difficult long-
term project. As we noted in the conclusion to our 1989 pilot study, we have
consistently found practitioners in the mental health disciplines to be largely
unaware of many of the important issues surrounding their patient records. But we
have also consistently found them to be eager to address those issues and explore
strategies for improving their work.

Chapter 7

New Developments: 1992 to 1994

Since the publication of the first edition of this book in 1992, researchers have been active in exploring mental health records issues and, more generally, the language of the mental health professions. In this chapter we offer a representative sampling of this recent scholarship, presenting updates and other pertinent new material. We have arranged the material in this chapter topically, according to applicable key issue headings in the introduction and chapters 2 through 6.

THE MENTAL HEALTH PICTURE TODAY:
AN UPDATED SKETCH

Until recently, most estimates of the prevalence of mental illness (including ours) have been based on the ECA program. The ECA studies, which we described and used a basis for raising questions about *DSM* validity and reliability in chapter 4, have been superseded by the National Comorbidity Study (NCS). This 18-month study completed in 1992 sought to measure the prevalence of 14 of the most common mental disorders described in *DSM–III–R*, as well as measure the prevalence of comorbidity—that is, persons suffering from multiple disorders concurrently. Unlike the ECA program, which interviewed adults in five areas of the United States, the NCS had 8,098 respondents between the ages of 15 and 54 from the 48 contiguous states (Kessler et al., 1994). The NCS project, with a stratified multistage area probability sample and a lower age limit for interviewees than the ECA project, reflected a growing concern about mental illness in adolescents and a desire to construct a more representative picture of mental illness today.

An Associated Press ("Half of Americans," 1994) story comments on the NCS project and quotes Dr. Harold Pincus, director of research for the APA, as saying that "the new study is likely 'to reflect reality more accurately' than any previous one" (1994). Trained interviewers in the NCS used a modified form of the Composite International Diagnostic Interview, which has high diagnostic validity, interrater and test–retest reliabilities, and is a refined version of the DIS used in the ECA. Interviewers determined lifetime occurences of mental illness, as well as episodes within the 12 months prior to the interview. In the introduction to our first edition, we said that current statistics on the prevalence of mental illness in our culture may indicate the tip of an iceberg; the NCS confirms this claim and reveals more than the tip. Kessler and colleagues (1994) summarized the survey findings as follows:

> Nearly 50% of respondents reported at least one lifetime disorder, and close to 30% reported at least one 12-month disorder. The most common disorders were major depressive episode, alcohol dependence, social phobia, and simple phobia. More than half of all lifetime disorders occurred in the 14% of the population who had a history of three or more comorbid disorders. Less than 40% of those with a lifetime disorder had ever received professional treatment, and less than 20% of those with a recent disorder had been in treatment during the past 12 months. ... The prevalence of psychiatric disorders is greater than previously thought to be the case. ... Even among people with a lifetime history of three or more comorbid disorders, the proportion who ever obtain specialty sector mental health treatment is less than 50%. These results argue for the importance of more outreach and more research on barriers to professional help-seeking. (p. 8)

That half of the population is now predicted to experience mental illness at some point during their lives does not mean, of course, that all of those affected will actually seek treatment. Many illnesses are mild, and many people learn to cope with their disorders or "cure" themselves. The newly discovered large number of people at higher risk because of comorbidity who are not receiving treatment, however, and the authors' call for more outreach and research on barriers to professional help-seeking suggest that even larger numbers of people than we had originally noted are likely to enter mental health care delivery systems in the future, and with their entrance will come even larger numbers of and reliances on mental health records than we had predicted.

The NCS also confirms or places in sharper relief a number of features from earlier prevalence studies we cited. Kessler and colleagues (1994) reported that depression and alcohol abuse are the most common lifetime psychiatric disorders (17.1% and 14.1%, respectively), men are more likely to have substance abuse disorders and antisocial personality disorders than women, women are more likely to have affective and anxiety disorders than men, and lifetime disorders tend to be multiple (e.g., 79% of those who had a disorder were comorbid). The impact of multiple disorders is indicated by the fact that the 14% of the population that had three or more lifetime disorders accounted for 58.9% of those reporting disorders in the last 12 months and 89.5% of those reporting severe disorders in the last 12 months.

These predictions of increased prevalence of mental disorders and the probability of more people seeking treatment for them come at a time when health care costs are rising almost uncontrollably, and becoming the focus of serious concern among legislators and the public alike. In the introduction, we noted that public perceptions about mental illness had shifted dramatically during the last two decades, from a tendency to believe that mental disorders were weaknesses of will to an acceptance of them as illnesses, but we also noted that insurance companies were reducing coverage for treatment, and could do so because of the relative imprecision of mental health diagnosis. In an article linking the rising costs of health care and the validity of mental disorders as illnesses, Vatz and Weinberg (1992) reported that

> psychiatry continues to try to medicalize the unavoidable problems of life in a modern, complex society. ... Thomas Szasz, psychiatry's foremost critic, has argued for over 30 years that most of what is incorrectly called "mental illness" simply constitutes problems in living, or freely chosen deviant behavior. Illness, Dr. Szasz argues, is exclusively "a condition of the body ... a structural or functional abnormality of cells, tissues, organs or bodies." (p. A15)

The authors also identified rising costs of treatment as a central force behind this criticism, and reimbursements by third-party payors such as insurance companies as an equally key factor. They close by saying that "the economics of 'mental illness' may force a closer examination of the way we interpret many problems in living" (p. A15). We see these remarks as constituting additional evidence supporting our contention that external factors profoundly shape mental health records, even what is defined as illness in the mental health professions' central document, the *DSM*.

DSM–IV (1994) was published since the release of our first edition, and contains a myriad of revisions that are summarized in an 18-page appendix, "Annotated Listing of Changes in *DSM–IV*." Changes include fuller definitions of some disorders, changes in diagnostic criteria, a listing of 8 disorders deleted or subsumed into other categories, 13 new disorders (a net expansion of 5), and 16 major categories, some renamed, rather than the 15 of *DSM–III–R* (e.g., "Behavioral Eating Disorders" is now a major category rather than a subcategory of "Disorders Usually First Diagnosed in Infancy, Childhood, or Adolescence"). The name of one major category has been changed from "Organic Mental Disorders" to "Delirium, Dementia, and Amnestic and Other Cognitive Disorders." This change, we think, was likely made in response to arguments such as those described by Vatz and Weinberg (1992). "Organic" raised the issue of etiology, and whether other disorders have such a cause. By implication, the chain of questioning can be extended: If a disorder does not have an organic cause, is it a disorder or simply a problem of living in today's world or a chosen deviant behavior? The change in category name and the explanation for it attempt to preempt these kinds of questions: "In *DSM–III–R*, these disorders were included in the Organic Mental Disorders section. The term 'organic mental disorder' has been eliminated from *DSM–IV* because it implies that the other disorders in the manual do not have an 'organic' component" (*DSM–IV*, p. 776). This sensitivity to the issue of whether a disorder is an illness if no organic cause can be found was present in previous *DSM* editions, but to a much lesser degree. As preamble to the definition of mental disorder in the previous edition, the authors caution that "although this manual provides a classification of mental disorders, no definition adequately specifies precise boundaries for the concept of 'mental disorder' (this is also true for such concepts as physical disorder and mental physical health)" (p. xxii). An increased sensitivity to this question in the current edition is evidenced by the change in category title, and by increased rhetorical sharpness in the preamble to the definition of mental disorder:

> Although this volume is titled the *Diagnostic and Statistical Manual of Mental Disorders*, the term *mental disorder* unfortunately implies a distinction between "mental" disorders and "physical" disorders that is a reductionistic anachronism of mind/body dualism. A compelling literature documents that there is much "physical" in mental disorders and much "mental" in physical disorders. The problem raised by the term "mental" disorders has been much clearer than its solution, and, unfortunately, the term persists in the title of *DSM–IV* because we have not found an appropriate substitute. (p. xxi)

DSM–IV thus responds to external pressures such as economics and the importance of third-party payors while continuing to shape the reality of mental illness and the records chronicling it. Although changes in the newest edition are numerous, the frailties of the *DSM* as a language system that we described in chapter 4 remain. We return to the *DSM* in more detail later in this chapter.

As economics and third-party payors continue to be important factors affecting mental health records, so too is litigation. The APA's draft (1990) of *Record Keeping Guidelines* was recently published in final form (1993). After a brief introduction which notes that the guidelines are not meant to preempt professional judgments, the first body-paragraph stresses that promoting quality of patient care is the principal purpose of mental health records. The next four paragraphs, however, describe purposes of records in relation to the psychologist; to institutional, financial, and legal requirements; to protection in the event of litigation; and to state and federal statutes. The final paragraph addresses the issue of confidentiality and the growing number of secondary readers of these records:

> Psychologists are justifiably concerned that, at times, record keeping information will be required to be disclosed against the wishes of the psychologist or client, and may be released to persons unqualified to interpret such records. These guidelines assume that no record is free from disclosure all of the time, regardless of the wishes of the client or the psychologist. (p. 985)

The roles that mental health records play in relation to state and federal statutes and civil litigation thus remain as integral as we noted in our first edition and are, in fact, coming to be more widely recognized.

Our original sketch of the mental health picture and the place of records within it has, therefore, not fundamentally changed. The primary differences are sharper lines of relief in that picture (or that the picture is now in a bit larger frame) and an even further-growing importance of patient records in it.

THE TAXONOMY OF RECORDS

Although we have not yet sought to identify other care-delivery systems than the five we describe in chapter 2, we did want to return briefly to our taxonomy of mental health records to reemphasize our point about the constantly unfolding complexity of mental health records in various delivery systems. We are currently conducting a long-term qualitative study of the written communication processes and practices of a single mental health team working in an MHU within a correctional institution. In the description in chapter 2 of the records written and read in the correctional model, we identified 11 documents comprising the total correctional record, one of which was the initial plans and progress notes written by a psychiatric nurse. Our current research has revealed that the situation is considerably more complex than we had thought. This particular document might be more accurately titled initial plans and initial progress notes; our description and rhetorical analysis of it is accurate, but we now know that there is another set of progress notes which are not "initial." Ongoing progress notes are written by psychiatric nurses; however, these notes also have sections written by psychologists, psychological assistants, and social workers. Furthermore, a psychological assessment differing in purpose, audience, and use from psychological evaluation or psychological assessment for parole is part of these ongoing progress notes. Our point here is not to create confusion but to emphasize that we continue to find new layers of complexity in our taxonomy, in much the same way that our entire project continues to reveal new layers of rhetorical complexity in mental health records.

BIAS AND SOCIAL CONSTRUCTION
IN DISCOURSE COMMUNITIES

In 1992 when the first edition of this book was in press, so too was Bazerman and Paradis' (1991) important collection *Textual Dynamics of the Professions,* which contains a seminal study on how *DSM–III* shapes reality in the mental health professions. McCarthy's contribution to that collection reports on her 2-year case study of "Dr. Page," a child psychiatrist, and how *DSM–III* shapes what she knows and writes about mental illness in her patient records—that is, how the *DSM* shapes the reality of mental health for this clinician and the discourse community to which she belongs. McCarthy described the central question in her project as "how does the *DSM–III* manual shape Dr. Page's diagnostic work: her information gathering, her analyses, and her writing? That is, what are the epistemological and textual consequences of *DSM–III*?" (p. 359). To answer this question, McCarthy applied methods of ethnographic research in her case study, using multiple sources of information (triangulation) about Dr. Page's clinical and writing practices: interviews with Page and the readers of her reports, discourse-based interviews, document analyses of Page's diagnostic evaluation reports, a log kept by Page about her data gathering practices, audiotapes of her composing and dictating reports, and personal observation. (McCarthy, as a participant/observer, was represented to Page's colleagues in the hospital as a "friend and co-researcher"; p. 363.)

McCarthy reported that *DSM–III* controlled the amount and kind of information that Dr. Page gathered about her patients. The author illustrated her point by describing the parental interview of one of Page's patients, and how the psychiatrist used the Kiddie/SADS interview schedule to gather information and carefully document the sources of that information. This highly structured interview is a collection of questions that directly elicit information about the various behaviors described in operationally defined criteria for *DSM* diagnoses of mental disorders. In other words, McCarthy found that the *DSM* controls what is important in relation to diagnosing mental disorders, and renders other information insignificant. McCarthy noted that the *DSM* also governed the evaluation of the information gathered during the interview. In Page's report, a diagnostic evaluation,

> six of ... eight headings in her evaluation ... reflect *DSM–III* assumptions about what counts as relevant information in defining mental disorder. These six headings all focus on the clinical features of the case and Dr. Page's sources of information about these features. Because *DSM–III* takes a descriptive approach to mental illness, the clinical features of the case are ... the *sin qua non* of diagnosis. (p. 368)

In a discourse-based interview, McCarthy asked the psychiatrist if she would be willing to delete the information-sources section of her diagnosis. Page said no, because this body of information enhances the reliability of her diagnosis (i.e., the diagnosis contained in the "conclusions and recommendations" section of her report is arrived at by applying the rules of diagnosis specified in *DSM–III*). McCarthy called *DSM–III* the "charter document" of psychiatry because it specifies what is significant and dictates how one interprets it. She explained her choice of charter document as metaphor:

> The charter document of a social or political group establishes an organizing framework that specifies what is significant and draws people's attention to certain rules and relationships. In other words the charter defines as authoritative certain ways of seeing and deflects attention from other ways. It thus stabilizes a particular reality and sets the terms of future discussions. (p. 359)

McCarthy offered a powerful argument for *DSM–III* as a charter document for the mental health community. This collection of operationally defined criteria for diagnosing mental disorders, and prescriptions for the very reasoning that leads to that diagnosing, shapes the reality of this discourse community. And it is the community itself that gives ascent to this reality. As McCarthy noted in the opening sentence of her essay, "In 1979, the 34,000 members of the American Psychiatric Association *voted to approve* the third edition of its *Diagnostic and Statistical Manual of Mental Disorders*" (p. 358; italics added).

BIAS: GENDER AND RACE

Hedges and Schwartz (1990) studied the influence of patient gender and race on diagnosis and length of stay in a psychiatric hospital. Their work, set in an inner-city hospital for acute psychiatric patients, examined records written between 1987 and 1988, and sought to determine if diagnosis, length of stay, gender, and race are related. The authors pointed out that their question was posed in the context of current practice favoring short-term (30 days or less) intervention and return to the community over long-term custodial approaches. In reviewing the literature on the influence of gender and race, they distinguished their study from those conducted previously by noting that most have focused on prevalence of treatment rather than hospital admission and length of stay. Because their study was set in the inner city, patients were generally of lower socioeconomic status, eliminating the variable of class. (This limits the study's generalizability but provides one important advantage. The authors cite research by Warheit, Holzer & Arey, 1975, correlating class and prevalence of mental disorders, and dismissing race as a major factor when sociodemographics are considered. Their own study, however, fortuitously controlled for socioeconomics.) Hedges and Schwartz's document sample included 579 discharge summaries of patients diagnosed as suffering from schizophrenia-paranoid type, schizophrenia-undifferentiated, depression, and bipolar disorders. The sample was divided quite evenly by gender (52.3% males) and race (49.6% non-White, with all but 3 being Black).

Results showed a lack of bivariate relationship between length of stay and race or gender, but there was a relationship between race and principal diagnosis. Although class was not a factor, 81.6% of Blacks' diagnoses were schizophrenia, whereas only 61.6% of Whites' were. An examination of the interaction of gender, diagnosis, and length of stay showed that women diagnosed as schizophrenic were likely to remain hospitalized longer than men with that diagnosis, whereas men diagnosed with depression and bipolar disorders had longer stays than women with that diagnosis. Adding race as a factor, "66% of Black women with diagnoses of schizophrenia remain[ed] in the institution for more than 25 days, as compared to 59% of White men, 56% of White women, and 49% of Black men" (p. 263). The authors concluded that, no matter how these findings are interpreted, gender and racial differences are a problem warranting further study. (A tacit assumption in the study was that all 579 diagnoses were accurate. No mention is made whether structured interviews were used in the process of diagnosing patients, or whether any tests of diagnostic validity were conducted. Hedges and Schwartz speculated that, if clinical differences exist among races and genders, more discriminating diagnoses are needed.)

A broader and more radical interrogation of the relationship between race and bias is taken up by Good (1992–1993) in a special collection of essays focusing on comorbidity of mood disorders and substance abuse among American Indians and Alaskan natives. Good's essay differs from others in the collection in that it is neither based on epidemiological research nor written by a clinician. Good focused on social origins of these problems, and how culture shapes psychiatric illness and substance abuse, to raise a range of fundamental questions about race, ethnicity, and psychiatric diagnosis. His argument is for interdisciplinary research on the relationship of culture and diagnosis, that advances in psychiatric epidemiology provide an opportunity for collaboration between clinicians and anthropologists on problems of diagnosis across U.S. subcultures with a focus on misdiagnosis in minority communities.

Good summarizes the history of *DSM*'s development through several editions, emphasizing the focus in *III* and *III–R* on framing disorders as discrete, nonoverlapping categories of symptom sets. This "neo-Kraepelinian" approach was a movement toward a medical model for mental illness, a model that claims theoretical neutrality and emphasizes descriptive symptom criteria that are universal (i.e., culturally blind). Good noted that this trend tended to "reify classical European ... ethnopsychological concepts" (p. 429) and ignore social context, overemphasizing the individual as the source of pathology. He offered evidence of possible problems related to this conceptual framework by citing studies that reexamine diagnoses or compare chart diagnoses with research diagnoses (produced by using structured interviews like the Schedule for Affective Disorders and Schizophrenia [SADS]): Mukherjee, Shukla, Woodle, Rosen, and Olarte (1983) found that examining the charts of 76 patients revealed high levels of misdiagnosis of schizophrenia for all patients, but even higher levels for minority patients (51% Whites, 86% Blacks, 83% Hispanics). Good also cited a study by Pavkov et al. (1989) that used SADS to rediagnose 313 patients, and applied regression analysis to the results: To be Black was predictive of schizophrenia as a diagnosis. Good did not deny clinician bias as the possible cause of misdiagnosis; instead, he explored additional, more radical explanations.

Clinician interviews of patients, whether structured or open, are conducted within social and cultural contexts that may have norms that constrain significant information necessary for accurate diagnosis. Good noted, for example, that asking questions about painful or shameful experiences is extremely inappropriate in the Flathead Indian community, and is likely to produce partial responses with obvious impacts on the accuracy of diagnoses. Even the efficacy ascribed to structured interviews like the DIS in producing diagnoses of high validity, what Good called "the gold standard" (p. 435), is called into question when the communication is cross-cultural. He raised additional questions about even more fundamental issues considered by members of the *DSM–IV* Task Force, which debated research by several cross-cultural research teams including Guaranaccia, Good, and Kleinman (1990). Considerable evidence supports the notion that *Ataques de nervios*, which combines symptoms of depression and anxiety and expresses them in a somatic idiom, is a culturally distinct syndrome among Puerto Ricans. The neo-Kraepelinian position presupposes that disorders are universal, that culture does not shape presenting symptoms. This apparently contradictory evidence potentially strikes at the very heart of the *DSM* and the biomedical model.

Good raised troubling questions about cultural bias that probe far deeper than issues of clinician bias. He even examined the *DSM–III Casebook* by Spitzer, Skodol, Gibbon, and Williams (1981), which is used to teach *DSM* multi-axial diagnosis through analysis of cases presented in narrative form. Good found the demographics of the imaginary patients in the scenarios to be predominantly professional or middle class, with only 11% identified as working class and only 1 of 87, "Emelio," implied to be ethnic. His suggestion is not that a larger number of ethnic names would somehow improve the collection. Rather, he pointed to an oversimplification and perhaps unwise emphasis on mental illness as universal and acultural in a book that he speculated may function as a rhetorically powerful recitation of disorder prototypes. He concluded that the questions and possible difficulties he raises should be viewed as opportunities for collaborative research by clinicians, epidemiologists, and anthropologists.

In response to the concerns described by Good and the research he cited, *DSM–IV* (1994) includes "Appendix I: Outline for Cultural Formulation and Glossary of Culture-Bound Syndromes." This seven-page addition, divided into two parts, provides suggestion for gathering and recording information on the patient's cultural identity and community, including communal explanations of the disorder, and on communication problems that may be caused by differences in culture and class between clinicians and patients. Among the 12 culture-bound syndromes described is *Ataque de nervios*. In addition, *DSM–IV* includes a section titled "Specific Culture, Age, and Gender Features" for each disorder.

BIAS: ACADEMIC AND SCIENTIFIC DISCOURSE

Earlier, we outlined differences between academic discourse, which tends to view language as a filter—as rhetorical, epistemic, and subjective or social—and scientific discourse, which tends to view language as a transparent windowpane—as arhetorical, reality-reporting, and objective. Here, we briefly illustrate the blurring of these two categories by Bromley (1991) as he instructed psychological counselors on improving scientific discourse (case reports) by applying a tool of academic discourse (discourse analysis). Bromley argued that case reports have a significant rhetorical components and therefore require that writers possess discourse knowledge to effectively persuade readers of their understanding of patients. Content knowledge (data) is of course also required but, argued Bromley, in itself not adequate to write a sound case report. Bromley also defined coherence and cohesion, how they function in a successful report, and how they can be established in a text. After a brief discussion of the composing process from a cognitive perspective, Bromley returned to the topic of coherence and discussed how the logic of substantive arguments imposes it. He advocated using Toulmin's approach to analyzing substantive arguments in case reports to improve the persuasive power of the text and especially to identify omissions that may be difficult for report readers to supply. Although Bromley separated case reports from psychological experiments by invoking distinctions between the qualitative and the quantitative, he did frame this particular mental health record in terms of academic rather than scientific discourse, blurring the distinctions we described in chapter 4.

EVEN MORE ON THE *DSM*

McCarthy and Gerring (1994) continued the work on *DSM* as a charter document that we discussed earlier by following the revision process that led to the publication of *DSM–IV*. In their 3-year study of revision, the authors analyzed the history of earlier revisions of the manual, the published accounts by Task Force leaders of the most recent revision, and the deliberations and other activities of one workgroup's revision process. Their study employed naturalistic research methods including interviews with Task Force leaders, work-group members, and clinicians not involved in the revision; observations of several work-group sessions; document analyses of all group writings related to the revision; and verifications of accuracy for all group members quoted.

The authors' history of earlier revisions sets the context for the most recent revision. The authors traced the ascendance of the medical model at the heart of *DSM–III* and subsequent editions, including struggles for theoretical dominance and the part that rhetoric plays in them, social perceptions of psychiatry as a sophisticated disciplinary subdivision of medicine, differentiations of psychiatry from other mental health professions, and consolidations of disciplinary control.

In analyzing the seven articles by Task Force members justifying a revision of the *DSM* only 7 years after the previous edition, the authors studied how those articles address key concerns about the revision: that it would disrupt research begun but not yet completed; that it would imply disciplinary uncertainty or, worse, an admission of inadequate research underlying earlier editions; and, adequate new data for substantive changes being unlikely, that it would be seen as tinkering or, even more cynically, financially motivated. McCarthy and Gerring found that Task Force members who authored articles responding to these concerns sought to persuade readers that the revision would have a broader empirical base than previous editions and, at the same time, that the broader empirical base existed because of the earlier editions and the research they enabled. In the first part of their response, then, Task Force members distance *DSM–IV* from its predecessors and, in the second part, they directly connect the new edition to its predecessors. The newest revision is cast as an important (and, by implication, necessary) advance without denigrating the earlier edition which made the advance possible. McCarthy and Gerring also noted that both of these strategies (distancing and connecting) are congenial to the neo-Kraepelinian view and help further the dominance of the biomedical model.

The authors studied the revision activities of the work-group assigned to eating disorders, and particularly focused on the group's deliberations about adding a new disorder, the Binge Eating Disorder. Of the five areas the group considered for revision, it was the addition of Behavioral Eating Disorder that generated the most controversy and required the most rhetorical negotiations among group members. In these negotiations, McCarthy and Gerring found several principles to be guiding the process, including a careful effort to preserve and promote the image of psychiatry as a mature and certain science through heavy emphasis on empirical data, a privileging of theory and research to enhance an image of professionalism, and a sensitivity to possible political, economic, and social ramifications if the disorder was added. The first two of these principles seem clear, but the third requires some specific examples. In the debate about adding the disorder, members of the group were concerned about the political impact of such an addition in terms of stigmatizing part of the obese population, and economic concerns were embodied in discussion of insurance companies' willingness to reimburse for treatment of such a disorder. The social emerged in concerns about professional image: Would the public see the addition as simply a move to broaden psychiatry's patient base?

McCarthy and Gerring provide an interesting perspective on the revision of the *DSM* while also providing an institutional analysis of psychiatry and an initial defining of its discursive practices. The authors summarize as follows:

> Our overall conclusion from this three-part study is that revision of the *DSM* manual functions less to change the text than to achieve the following three effects: (a) to further solidify the dominance of the biomedical model of mental disorder within psychiatry, (b) to maintain the position of psychiatry as *the* high-status profession among competing disciplines within the mental health field, and (c) to achieve acceptance of psychiatry as a mature, research-based specialty within medicine. (p. 149)

IMPROVING MENTAL HEALTH RECORDS: RESEARCH PRIORITIES

Several of the articles we cite in this chapter suggest research—for example, on issues of diagnostic validity and race or gender (Hedges & Schwartz, 1990; Pavkov et al., 1989; Warheit et al., 1975), and issues of diagnostic validity and race or ethnicity (Good, 1992–1993; Guaranaccia et al., 1990; Mukherjee et al., 1983). We find it interesting but not surprising that the research and the research priorities being suggested revolve around the *DSM* and its various editions. McCarthy's (1991) and McCarthy and Gerring's (1994) suggestions again revolve around the *DSM* and issues of social construction, discourse communities, discursive practices, and institutional analyses. The manual remains absolutely central to mental health care and problematic in its rhetorical and diagnostic frailties. It impacts mental health records in immediate ways (diagnoses are determined and reported according to its dictates) but also in other, more ultimate ways prior to acts of writing/reading those records. Other research in the field critiques premises that precede assumptions on which *DSM* is built. Hoagwood's (1993) critique of the psychological construction of anxiety disorders from the position of poststructuralism and historicism suggests a new construction of disorders from, among other things, the perspective of subject positions rather than self as unitary. Two articles (APA, 1993; Bromley, 1991) that we consider here that directly address writing/reading issues are instructional rather than analytic. We spoke of the need for interdisciplinary approaches to instruction in our first edition, and Bromley is a move in that direction. Good's suggestion that epidemiologists, clinicians, and anthropologists collaborate is also a move toward interdisciplinarity in realms of research. Interest in our topic obviously does cross disciplines, as indicated by the very distribution of reviews of the first edition of this book: half appeared in rhetoric journals and half in mental health journals.

What we find most unchanged since 1992 is our own reaction to what we have learned, and continue to learn, about the relationships among rhetoric, mental health records, and the various forces and contexts that shape them. We continue to be fascinated by these relationships, and amazed each time we rediscover that while the layers of complexity wrapping the writing and reading of these records are apparently endless, all roads inevitably lead to the *DSM*.

Postscript

It seems as though we have created a whole industry called Patient Records. Where will it end? Maybe, just maybe, it will end when the buildings that store all of these records begin to collapse one by one from the sheer weight of the paper involved. When that happens, there'll be an earthquake measuring about 13 on the Richter Scale. Oceans will rise, but will quickly dry up from the records absorbing all the water. Cities will be buried, not by rubble, but by records. The weight of all the now-wet patient records will cause all of the remaining buildings to collapse, and people will be suffocated by wet, drying patient records. As winds from tidal waves begin to blow, they'll carry the records to faraway places. And then—well, then the records will no longer be confidential. As they dry, they'll be read by everyone left on the planet. Everyone will read them and will know what was in them. The very purpose of records will cease to exist. People will laugh and laugh at the ridiculous, absurd, CYA graffiti that mental health professionals have been writing about their patients, all in the name of confidentiality. The secrets will be secrets no more. Or, maybe the records will all just be computerized, and the weight of all the hardware and software and modems and stuff will cause the same kind of catastrophe ...

—John C. Wolfe, PhD
Clinical Psychologist and Administrator

References and Bibliography

Allen, R.H., Webb, L.J., & Gold, R.S. (1980). Validity of problem-oriented record system for evaluating treatment outcome. *Psychological Reports, 47,* 303–306.

American Psychiatric Association. (1952). *Diagnostic and statistical manual of mental disorders.* Washington, DC: Author.

American Psychiatric Association. (1980). *Diagnostic and statistical manual of mental disorders* (3rd ed.). Washington, DC: Author.

American Psychiatric Association. (1987). *Diagnostic and statistical manual of mental disorders* (3rd ed. rev.). Washington, DC: Author.

American Psychiatric Association. (1994). *Diagnostic and statistical manual of mental disorders* (4th ed.). Washington, DC: Author.

American Psychological Association. (1990). *Record keeping guidelines* (3rd draft). Washington, DC: Author, Committee on Professional Practice and Standards.

American Psychological Association. (1993). Record keeping guidelines. *American Psychologist, 48,* 984–986.

American Psychological Association. (1977). *Standards for providers of psychological services.* Washington, DC: Author.

Appelbaum, S.A. (1970). Science and persuasion in the psychological test report. *Journal of School Psychology, 35,* 349–355.

Association for the Psychiatric Treatment of Offenders. (1971). The court and the expert: Writing reports. *APTO Monographs,* No.3.

Bagnato, S.J. (1980). The efficacy of diagnostic reports as individualized guides to prescriptive goal planning. *Exceptional Children, 46,* 554–557.

Barnett, G.O., & Winickoff, R.N. (1990). Quality assurance and computer-based patient records. *American Journal of Public Health, 80,* 527–528.

Bass, A. (1990, November 21). *Alcohol, drug abuse linked to mental illness.* [Nationally syndicated newspaper column].

Bazerman, C., & Paradis, J. (Eds.). (1991). *Textual dynamics of the professions: Historical and contemporary studies of writing in professional communities.* Madison: University of Wisconsin Press.

Bellak, L. (1959). Psychological test reporting: A problem in communication between psychologists and psychiatrists. Introduction: The scope of the problem. *Journal of Nervous Mental Disorders, 129,* 76–77.

Bender, K.J. (1990). *Psychiatric medications: A guide for mental health professionals.* Newbury Park, CA: Sage.

Biagi, E. (1977). The social work stake in problem-oriented recording. *Social Work in Health Care, 3,* 211–221.

Bjork, R., & Oye, R.K. (1983, February). Writing courses in American medical schools. *Journal of Medical Education, 112,* 116.

Bledstein, B. (1977). *The culture of professionalism.* New York: Norton.

Bollinger, R.A. (1985). Differences between pastoral counseling and psychotherapy. *Bulletin of the Menninger Clinic, 49,* 371–386.

Borus, J.F., Howes, M.J., Devins, N.P., Rosenberg, R., & Livingston, W.W. (1988). Primary health care providers' recognition and diagnosis of mental disorders in their patients. *General Hospital Psychiatry, 10,* 317–321.

Boyd, J.H., Burke, J.D., Gruenberg, E., Holzer, C.E., & Rae, D.S. (1984). Exclusion criteria of DSM–III. *Archives of General Psychiatry, 41,* 983–989.

Brandt, H.M., & Giebink, J.W. (1968). Concreteness and congruence in psychologists' reports to teachers. *Psychology in the Schools, 5,* 87–89.

Bromley, D.B. (1991). Academic contributions to psychological counselling. 2. Discourse analysis and the formulation of case-reports. *Counselling Psychology Quarterly, 4,* 75–89.

Brower, R. (1959). *On translation.* Cambridge, MA: Harvard University Press.

Bruffee, K.A. (1986). Social construction: Language and the authority of knowledge. *College English, 48,* 773–790.

Carlton, S.B. (1990, May). *Ethical subjectivity and discursive practice.* Paper presented at the annual conference of the Rhetoric Society of America, Arlington, TX.

Christie, K.A., Burke, J.D., Regier, D.A., et al. (1988). Epidemiologic evidence for early onset of mental disorders and higher risk of drug abuse in young adults. *American Journal of Psychiatry, 145,* 971–975.

Cuadra, C.A., & Albaugh, W.P. (1956). Sources of ambiguity in psychological reports. *Journal of Clinical Psychology, 12,* 109–115.

Dailey, C.A. (1953). The practical utility of the clinical report. *Journal of Consulting Psychology, 17,* 297–302.

Dean, E.S. (1963). Writing psychiatric reports. *American Journal of Psychiatry, 119,* 759–762.

Donnelly, W.J. (1988). Righting the medical record: Transforming chronicle into story. *Journal of the American Medical Association, 260,* 823–825.

Eaton, W.W., Holzer, C.E., Von Korff, M., Anthony, J.C., & Helzer, J.E. (1984). The design of the Epidemiologic Catchment Area surveys. *Archives of General Psychiatry, 41,* 942–948.

Eaton, W.W., Kramer, M., et al. (1989). The incidence of specific DIS/DSM–III mental disorders: data from the NIMH Epidemiologic Catchment Area Program. *Acta Psychiatric Scandanavia, 79,* 163–178.

Eberst, N.D., & Genshaft, J. (1984). Differences in school psychological report writing as a function of doctoral vs. non-doctoral training. *Psychology in the Schools, 21,* 78–82.

Elbow, P. (1991). Reflections on academic discourse: How it relates to freshmen and colleagues. *College English, 53,* 135–155.

Feifel, H. (1959). Psychological test reporting: A problem in communication between psychologists and psychiatrists. Psychological test report: A communication between psychologist and psychiatrist. *Journal of Nervous Mental Disorders, 129,* 77–81.

Fish, S. (1989). Withholding the missing portion: Psychoanalysis and rhetoric. In S. Fish (Ed.), *Doing what comes naturally: Change, rhetoric, and the practice of theory in literary and legal studies* (pp. 525–554). Durham, NC: Duke University Press.

Foster, A. (1951). Writing psychological reports. *Journal of Clinical Psychology, 7,* 195.

Fourth annual guide to better mental care. (1990, December 25–31). [Special Issue]. *PortFolio Magazine.*

Freed, E.X. (1975). The psychologist and the problem-oriented record. *New Jersey Psychologist, 25,* 9–10.

Freedman, D.X. (1984). Psychiatric epidemiology counts. *Archives of General Psychiatry, 41,* 931–933.

Garfield, S.L., Heine, R.W., & Leventhal, M. (1954). An evaluation of psychological reports in a clinical setting. *Journal of Consulting Psychology, 18,* 281–286.

Garrick, T.R., & Stotland, N.L. (1982). How to write a psychiatric consultation. *American Journal of Psychiatry, 139,* 849–855.

Good, B.J. (1992–1993). Culture, diagnosis, and comorbidity. *Culture, Medicine, and Psychiatry, 16,* 427–446.

Grant, R.L. (1979). The problem-oriented system and record keeping in the behavioral therapies. *Journal of Community Psychology, 7,* 53–59.

Grant, R., & Maletzky, B. (1972). Application of the Weed system to psychiatric records. *Psychiatry in Medicine, 3,* 119–129.

Grayson, H.M., & Tolman, R.S. (1950). A semantic study of concepts of clinical psychologists and psychiatrists. *Journal of Abnormal Social Psychology, 45,* 216–232.

Grounds, A. (1987). On describing mental states. *British Journal of Medical Psychology, 60,* 305–311.

Guaranaccia, P.J., Good, B.J., & Kleinman, A. (1990). A critical review of epidemiological studies of Puerto Rican mental health. *American Journal of Psychiatry, 147,* 1149–1456.

Haber, J. (1978). The problem-oriented record in psychiatry. *Issues in Mental Health Nursing, 1,* 91–102.

Half of Americans face mental illness some time, study says. (1994, January 14). *Associated Press.*

Hammond, K.R., & Allen, J.M. (1953). *Writing clinical reports.* New York: Prentice-Hall.

Hedges, R.H., & Schwartz, M.D. (1990). The influence of sex and race on psychiatric diagnoses and length of stay in acute psychiatric hospitalization. *International Review of Modern Sociology, 20,* 253–266.

Hoagwood, K. (1993). Poststructuralist historicism and the psychological construction of anxiety disorders. *The Journal of Psychology, 127,* 105–122.

Hoffman, B.F. (1986). How to write a psychiatric report for litigation following a personal injury. *American Journal of Psychiatry, 143,* 164–169.

Hollis, J.W., & Donn, P.A. (1979). *Psychological report writing: Theory and practice.* Muncie, IN: Accelerated Development.

Holton, G. (1965). *Science and culture: A study of cohesive and disjunctive forces.* Boston: Houghton.

Holzberg, J.D., Alessi, S.L., & Wexler, M. (1951). Psychological case reporting at psychiatric staff conferences. *Journal of Consulting Psychology, 15,* 425–429.

Horner, W.B. (1988). *Rhetoric in the classical tradition.* New York: St. Martin's.

Huber, J.T. (1961). *Report writing in psychology and psychiatry.* New York: Harper.

Joint Commission on Accreditation of Hospitals. (1984). *Consolidated standards manual, 1985.* Chicago: Author.

Judd, L.L. (1990). Putting mental health on the nation's health agenda. *Hospital and Community Psychology, 41.*

Karno, M., Golding, J.M., Sorenson, S.B., & Burnam, M.A. (1988). The epidemiology of obsessive-complsive disorder in five US communities. *Archives of General Psychiatry, 45,* 1094–1099.

Katz, R.C., & Woolley, F.R. (1975). Improving patient records through problem orientation. *Behavior Therapy, 6,* 119–124.

Kazdin, A.E., & Cole, P.M. (1981). Attitudes and labeling biases toward modification: The effects of labels, content and jargon. *Behavior Therapy, 12,* 56–58.

Kessler, R., McGonagle, K.A., Zhao, S., Nelson, C.B., Hughes, M., Eshleman, S., Wittchen, H., & Kendler, K.S. (1994). Lifetime and 12-month prevalence of *DSM–III–R* psychiatric disorders in the United States. *Archives of General Psychiatry, 51,* 8–19.

Kinneavy, J.L. (1971). *A theory of discourse.* Englewood Cliffs, NJ: Prentice-Hall.

Klopfer, W.G. (1959). Psychological test reporting: A problem in communication between psychologists and psychiatrists. The psychological report as a problem in interdisciplinary communication. *Journal of Nervous Mental Disorders, 129,* 86–88.

Klopfer, W.G. (1960). *The psychological report.* New York: Grune & Stratton.

Koss, M.P. (1990). The women's mental health research agenda: Violence against women. *American Psychologist, 45,* 374–380.

Kuhn, T.S. (1970). *The structure of scientific revolutions* (2nd ed.). Chicago: University of Chicago Press. (Original work published 1962)

Lacey, H.M., & Ross, A.O. (1964). Multidisciplinary views on psychological reports in child guidance clinics. *Journal of Clinical Psychology, 20,* 522–526.

Lacks, P.B., Horton, M.M., & Owen, J.D. (1969). A more meaningful and practical approach to psychological reports. *Journal of Clinical Psychology, 25,* 383–386.

Lanier, B. (1984, March 19). My patients fill in their own medical charts. *Medical Economics,* pp. 189–197.

Lanyon, R.I. (1986). Psychological assessment procedures in court-related settings. *Professional Psychology: Research and Practice, 17,* 260–268.

Lodge, G.T. (1953). How to write a psychological report. *Journal of Clinical Psychology, 9,* 400–402.

Mair, D., & Radovich, J. (1987). Developing industrial cases for technical writing on campus. *Journal of Advanced Composition*, *6*, 89–96.

Mair, D.C., & Reynolds, J.F. (1988). Writing mental health records, part II. *Journal of the Radix Teachers Association*, *1*, 13–14.

Majeski, T. (1991, June). Gay male teens suicide-prone. *Knight-Ridder News Service*.

Mandler, G., & Kessen, W. (1959). *The language of psychology*. New York: Wiley.

Martin, W.T. (1972). *Writing psychological reports*. Springfield, IL: Charles C. Thomas.

Masson, J.M. (1984). *The assault on truth*. New York: Farrar, Straus & Giroux.

Matalene, C.B. (Ed.). (1989). *Worlds of writing: Teaching and learning in discourse communities of work*. New York: Random House.

Matarazzo, J.D. (1990). Psychological assessment versus psychological testing. *American Psychologist*, *45*, 999–1017.

McCarthy, L.P. (1991). A psychiatrist using *DSM–III*: The influence of a charter document in psychiatry. In C. Bazerman & J. Paradis (Eds.), *Textual dynamics of the professions: Historical and contemporary studies of writing in professional communities* (pp. 358–378) .Madison: University of Wisconsin Press.

McCarthy, L.P., & Gerring, J.P. (1994). Revising psychiatry's charter document *DSM–IV*. *Written Communication*, *11*, 147–192.

McGrath, E., Kelta, G.P., Strickland, B.R., & Russo, N.F. (Eds.). (1990). *Women and depression: Risk factors and treatment issues* (Final Report of the APA's National Task Force on Women and Depression). Washington, DC: American Psychological Association.

Meredith, R.L., & Bair, S.L. (1990). Computer-generated client record keeping. *Register Report*, *16*, 15–19.

Merton, R. (1973). *The sociology of science*. Chicago: Univeristy of Chicago Press.

Merton, R. (1987). Three fragments from a sociologist's notebooks: Establishing the phenomenon, specified ignorance, and strategic research materials. *Annual Review of Sociology*, *13*, 1–28.

Miller, E. (1976). Growing "weeds": A problem-oriented approach to patient records in clinical psychology. *Bulletin of the British Psychological Society*, *29*, 359–362.

Morrow, R.S. (1954). The diagnostic psychological report. *Psychiatric Quarterly Supplement*, *28*, 102–110.

Mukherjee, S., Shukla, S., Woodle, J., Rosen, A.M., & Olarte, S. (1983). Misdiagnosis of schizophrenia in bipolar patients: A multiethnic comparison. *American Journal of Psychiatry*, *140*, 1571–1574.

Myers, J.K., Weissman, M.M., Tischler, G.L., Holzer, C.E., & Leaf, P.J. (1984). Six-month prevalence of psychiatric disorders in three communities. *Archives of General Psychiatry*, *41*, 959–967.

National Institute of Mental Health. (1988). *Media advisory: Report on the mental health of Americans published in pscyhiatric journal*. Rockville, MD: Author.

National Institute on Drug Abuse. (1989). *Overview of selected drug trends*. Rockville, MD: Author.

Neel, J. (1988). *Plato, Derrida, and writing*. Carbondale, IL: Southern Illinois University Press.

Odell, L., & Goswami, D. (1982). Writing in a non-academic setting. *Research in the Teaching of English*, *16*, 201–223.

Odell, L., & Goswami, D. (Eds.). (1985). *Writing in nonacademic settings*. New York: Guilford.

Pagano, M.P., & Mair, D. (1986). Writing medical records. *Journal of Technical Writing and Communication*, *16*, 331–341.

Pate, J.L. (1991, January 27). Soul wounds: War casualties include emotional harm. *Virginian Pilot/Ledger Star*, p. A3.

Pavkov, T.W., Lewis, D.A., & Lyons, J.S. (1989). Psychiatric diagnosis and racial bias: An empirical investigation. *Professional Psychology: Research and Practice*, *20*, 364–368.

Perr, I.N. (1984). Medical and legal problems in psychiatric coding under the DSM and ICD systems. *American Journal of Psychiatry*, *141*, 418–420.

Polanyi, M. (1964). *Science, faith and society*. Chicago: University of Chicago Press.

Popper, K. (1963). *Conjectures and refutations: The growth of scientific knowledge*. New York: Basic Books.

Psychiatric hospitals: Losing out in the new world order of insurance. (1991, April 22). *Virginian Pilot/Ledger Star Business Weekly*, p. 17.

Raymo, C. (1989, February 27). Just the facts, Ma'am. *Boston Globe*, p. 26.

Reeves, C. (1990). Establishing a phenomenon: The rhetoric of early medical reports on AIDS. *Written Communication, 7*, 393–416.

Regier, D.A., Boyd, J.H., Burke, J.D., Rae, D.S., & Myers, J.K. (1988). One-month prevalence of mental disorders in the United States. *Archives of General Psychiatry, 45*, 977–986.

Regier, D.A., Myers, J.K., Kramer, M., Robins, L.N., & Blazer, D.G. (1984). The NIMH Epidemiologic Catchment Area program. *Archives of General Psychiatry, 41*, 934–941.

Reynolds, J.F., & Mair, D. (1989a). Patient records in the mental health disciplines. *Journal of Technical Writing and Communication, 19*, 245–254.

Reynolds, J.F., & Mair, D.C. (1989b). Writing mental health records, part III. *Journal of the Radix Teachers Association, 2*, 9–11.

Robins, L.N., & Helzer, J.E. (1986). Diagnosis and clinical assessment: The current state of psychiatric diagnosis. *Annual Review of Psychology, 37*, 409–432.

Robins, L.N., Helzer, J.E., Weissman, M.M., Orvaschel, H., Gruenberg, E., & Burke, J.D. (1984). Lifetime prevalence of specific psychiatric disorders in three sites. *Archives of General Psychiatry, 41*, 949–958.

Rosenthal, A.M. (1990, November 24). *Doing no favors for the homeless.* [Nationally syndicated newspaper column].

Rossi, P.H. (1990). The old homeless and the new homelessness in historical perspective. *American Psychologist, 45*, 954–959.

Rucker, C.N. (1967). Technical language in the school psychologists' reports. *Psychology in the Schools, 4*, 146–150.

Ryback, R.S. (1974). *The problem-oriented record in psychiatry and mental health care.* New York: Grune & Stratton.

Ryback, R.S., & Gardner, S.J. (1973). Problem formulation: The problem-oriented record. *American Journal of Psychiatry, 130*, 312–316.

Ryback, R.S., Longabaugh, R., & Fowler, D.R. (1981). *The problem-oriented record in psychiatry and mental health care.* New York: Grune and Stratton.

Salvagno, M., & Teglasi, H. (1987). Teacher perceptions of different types of information in psychological reports. *Journal of School Psychology, 25*, 415–424.

Sargent, H.D. (1951). Psychological test reporting: An experiment in communication. *Bulletin of the Menninger Clinic, 15*, 175–186.

Schindler, F., Berren, M.R., Hannah, M.T., Beigel, A., & Santiago, J.M. (1987). How the public perceives psychiatrists, psychologists, nonpsychiatric physicians, and members of the clergy. *Professional Psychology: Research and Practice, 18*, 371–376.

Scholes, R. (1991). An end to hypocriticism. *South Central Review, 8*, 1–13.

Shapiro, S., Skinner, E.A., Kessler, L.G., Von Korff, M., & German, P.S. (1984). Utilization of health and mental health services. *Archives of General Psychiatry, 41*, 971–978.

Shively, J.J., & Smith, A.E. (1969). Understanding the psychological report. *Psychology in the Schools, 6*, 272–273.

Siegel, C., & Fischer, S.K. (Eds.). (1981). *Psychiatric records in mental health care.* New York: Brunner/Mazel.

6% of teens say they have tried suicide. (1991, April 4). *Associated Press.*

Sontag, S. (1988). *AIDS and its metaphors.* New York: Farrar, Straus & Giroux.

Soreff, S., Gulkin, T., & Pike, J.G. (1990). The evolving clinical chart: How it reflects and influences psychiatric and medical practice and the quality of care. *Psychiatric Clinics of North America, 13*, 127–133.

Spitzer, R.L., Skodol, A.E., Gibbon, M., & Williams, J.B.W. (1981). *DSM-III casebook.* Washington, DC: American Psychiatric Association.

Strachey, J. (Trans. and Ed.). (1966). *The complete introductory lectures on psychoanalysis by Sigmund Freud.* New York: Norton.

Steele, C.M., & Josephs, R.A. (1990). Alcohol myopia: Its prized and dangerous effects. *American Psychologist, 45*, 921–933.

Sturm, I.E. (1987). The psychologist in the problem-oriented record (POR). *Professional Psychology: Research and Practice, 18*, 155–158.

Tallent, N. (1956). An approach to the improvement of clinical psychological reports. *Journal of Clinical Psychology, 12*, 103–109.

Tallent, N. (1976). *Psychological report writing*. Englewood Cliffs, NJ: Prentice-Hall.

Tallent, N., & Reiss, W.J. (1959a). Multidisciplinary views on the preparation of written clinical psychological reports: I. Spontaneous suggestions for content. *Journal of Clinical Psychology, 15,* 218–221.

Tallent, N., & Reiss, W.J. (1959b). Multidisciplinary views on the preparation of written clinical psychological reports: II. Acceptability of certain common content variables and styles of expression. *Journal of Clinical Psychology, 15,* 273–274.

Tallent, N., & Reiss, W.J. (1959c). Multidisciplinary views on the preparation of written clinical psychological reports: III. The trouble with psychological reports. *Journal of Clinical Psychology, 15,* 444–446.

Taylor, J.L., & Teicher, A. (1946). A clinical approach to reporting psychological test data. *Journal of Clinical Psychology, 2,* 323–332.

U.S. Department of Health and Human Services. (1990, December 19). *HHS News*, pp. 1–5.

Van Vort, W., & Mattson, M.R. (1989). A strategy for enhancing the clinical utility of the psychiatric record. *Hospital and Community Psychiatry, 40,* 407–409.

Vatz, R.E., & Weinberg, L.S. (1992, January 17). Insuring the—so-called—mentally ill. *Virginian Pilot/Ledger Star,* p. A15.

Vitanza, V.J. (1987). Notes towards historiographies of rhetorics; or the rhetorics of the histories of rhetorics: Traditional, revisionary, and sub/versive. *Pre/Text, 8,* 63–125.

Warheit, G.J., Holzer, C.E., & Arey, S.A. (1975). Race and mental illness: An epidemiologic update. *Journal of Health and Social Behavior, 16,* 243–256.

Webb, L.J., Gold, R.S., Howes-Coleman, K., Holley, M.B., Reck, J., & Trusch, H. (1980). Reliability of a problem-oriented record system approach to the evaluation of treatment outcome. *Psychological Reports, 46,* 452–454.

Weed, L.L. (1968). Medical records that guide and teach. *New England Journal of Medicine, 278,* 593–600.

Weed, L.L. (1969). *Medical records, medical education, and patient care*. Cleveland, OH: Case Western Reserve University Press.

Weed, L.L. (1971). *Medical records, medical education, and patient care: The problem-oriented record as a basic tool*. Chicago: Year Book Medical Publishers.

Welch, K.E. (1987). Ideology and freshman textbook production: The place of theory in writing pedagogy. *College Composition and Communication, 38,* 269–282.

Wiener, J. (1985). Teachers' comprehension of psychological reports. *Psychology in the Schools, 22,* 60–64.

Wiener, J. (1987). Factors affecting educators' comprehension of psychological reports. *Psychology in the Schools, 24,* 116–126.

Wiener, J., & Kohler, S. (1986). Parents' comprehension of psychological reports. *Psychology in the Schools, 23,* 265–270.

Williams, S., Dixen, J, Calhoun, J.S., & Moss, R.A. (1982). Psychological report writing: Assessment and training of correctional personnel. *International Journal of Offender Therapy and Comparative Criminology, 26,* 126–132.

Woods, D. (1981). Good English is good medicine. *Canadian Medical Association Journal, 15,* 624.

Young, J.L., & Griffith, E.E.H. (1989). The development and practice of pastoral counseling. *Hospital and Community Psychiatry, 40,* 271–276.

Index

About the Authors

John Frederick Reynolds is Professor of English and Director of Language and Literacy at the City College of the City University of New York (CUNY), where he teaches a variety of undergraduate and graduate writing courses. He holds BA and MA degrees in speech communication and English from Midwestern (Texas) State University, and a PhD in composition studies from the University of Oklahoma. His research has been published in the *Journal of Advanced Composition*, the *Journal of Technical Writing and Communication*, the *Rhetoric Society Quarterly*, the *Technical Communication Quarterly*, and the *Computer-Assisted Composition Journal*, among others. He was previously Director of Professional Writing at Old Dominion University in Norfolk, Virginia, where much of his work focused on the writing and reading problems of adults working in highly specialized professions. Earlier he held positions in private school administration and corporate communications. He has been a consultant to NASA, the Boeing Company, and Norfolk Southern Corporation. He is also the author/editor of *Rhetorical Memory and Delivery: Classical Concepts for Contemporary Composition and Communication; Rhetoric, Cultural Studies, and Literacy: Selected Papers from the 1994 Conference of the Rhetoric Society of America*; and *Professional Writing in Context: Lessons from Teaching and Consulting in Worlds of Work*.

David Clare Mair is Associate Professor of English and Director of Composition and Technical Writing at the University of Oklahoma in Norman, Oklahoma, where he teaches courses in technical writing, composition theory, and research methods. He received his BA in English from the University of Missouri at Rolla, and his MA and PhD in English from the University of Utah. His research, much of which has focused on the composing processes of technical writers, has been published in the *Journal of Advanced Composition*, the *Journal of the Radix Teachers Association*, and the *Journal of Technical Writing and Communication*, among others. He is the coauthor of *Strategies for Technical Communication*. In addition to having previously worked as a technical writer in business and industry, Mair has been a consultant to a number of hospitals and engineering firms, and designed a 7-year plan for developing the writing skills of technical students at Lund University in Sweden. He has recently begun a long-term qualitative study of the written communication practices of a mental health care team working in a correctional setting.

Pamela Correia Fischer is a licensed psychologist in private practice in Oklahoma City, and an adjunct member of the faculties of the University of Oklahoma, Oklahoma City University, and the University of Oklahoma Health Sciences Center. She received her PhD in counseling psychology from Oklahoma State University. Additionally, she completed a 1-year clinical internship at the University of Kansas Medical School and a postdoctoral fellowship in medicine at the University of Oklahoma Health Sciences Center. Fischer, who has worked with adolescents, adults experiencing marriage and family problems, and patients suffering from eating disorders, chemical dependency, sexual problems, and AIDS, has nearly 25 years of experience as a provider of individual and group counseling and psychotherapy in school, clinic, and hospital settings. Her work has been presented at conventions of the American Psychological Association, and published in *Educational and Psychological Measurement* and the *Journal of Counseling and Development*.

About the Contributors

Kenneth J. Bender (PharmD, University of Southern California) is the author of *Psychiatric Medications* and a frequent contributor to *Psychiatric Times*. He maintains a psychiatric pharmacy practice at West Hills Hospital and Willow Springs Adolescent Residential Treatment Center in Reno, Nevada, where he is Director of Pharmacy Services. He previously held professorships in Pharmacy Practice at the University of Illinois and the University of Florida.

Robert C. Edwards (PhD, University of Oklahoma) is a retired clinical psychologist with the Oklahoma Department of Corrections. Previously he maintained private practices in Oklahoma City and Tulsa, Oklahoma, and served as clinical director of HCA Presbyterian Hospital's Center for Counseling and Psychotherapy in Oklahoma City.

Marcia K. Haynes (RNC, CHSA) is a correctional health services administrator with the Oklahoma Department of Corrections, for whom she previously served as the administrator of an 80-bed mental health unit that provided treatment for chronic and acutely psychotic offenders.

James L. Levenson (MD, University of Michigan) is Professor of Psychiatry, Medicine, and Surgery, and Chair of the Division of Consultation-Liaison Psychiatry at the Medical College of Virginia. He is an associate member of the Williamson Institute for Health Studies, chairman of the Hospital Ethics Committee, and a governor-appointed member of the Virginia Joint Legislative Subcommittee on AIDS. A consultant for both the National Institute of Mental Health and the Center for the Advancement of Health, he serves as a board examiner for the American Board of Psychiatry and Neurology, and was a member of APA's *DSM-IV* Subcommittee on Psychological Factors Affecting Physical Condition.

Lee Odell (PhD, University of Michigan) is Professor of Composition Theory and Research, and Associate Chair of the Department of Language, Literature, and Communication at Rensselaer Polytechnic Institute in Troy, New York. He has been a trustee of the National Council of Teachers of English Research Foundation, and currently chairs its Assembly for Research. He is the coauthor of *Evaluating*

Writing: Describing, Measuring, Judging and *Writing in Nonacademic Settings,* both of which are widely considered to be landmark works in composition studies. His most recent book is *Theory and Practice in the Teaching of Writing.*

Jennifer L. Ruhl (BBA, Georgia State University) is a former data services specialist for a large public hospital in Atlanta, Georgia.

Barbara A. Winstead (PhD, Harvard University) is a licensed clinical psychologist, Adjunct Associate Professor of Psychiatry and Behavioral Sciences at the Medical College of Hampton Roads, and Professor of Psychology at Old Dominion University in Norfolk, Virginia. She has been visiting professor of psychiatry at the University of Aukland, New Zealand, and a visiting professor of psychology at the University of Warsaw, Poland. She has published research analyzing the role of gender in the diagnosis and treatment of mental health problems.

John C. Wolfe (PhD, University of Oklahoma) is a board certified psychologist with more than 30 years of administrative experience in private, group, center, hospital, and government (NIAAA) settings. In addition to having held academic appointments at Bradley, St. Ambrose, and American Universities, and having been an APA fellow in 1981, he has been president of the American College of Mental Health Administrators, and has served as executive director of the National Council of Community Mental Health Centers, the chief operating officer of the National Psychiatric Institute and the Sheppard Pratt National Center for Human Development, and the chief executive officer of American Medical International and the AIDS Project of Los Angeles.

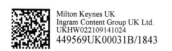